Dear
I hope this is
of some interest + use

First-time Father

I know you will

be a great Dad

much love

your Dad

Tony: To my mum and dad, who taught me about unconditional love; and to my five girls, who taught me about the importance of laughter, the reality of drama, and the need to put the toilet seat down.

Graeme: To Susan, with love and appreciation for our shared experience of parenting and grandparenting.

First-time Father
2nd edition

The essential guide for the new dad

Graeme Russell & Tony White

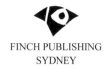

FINCH PUBLISHING
SYDNEY

First-time Father
This second edition first published in 2012 in Australia and New Zealand by
Finch Publishing Pty Limited. ABN 49 057 285 248, Suite 2207, 4 Daydream
Street, Warriewood, NSW, 2102, Australia.

14 13 12   8 7 6 5 4 3 2 1

National Library of Australia Cataloguing-in-Publication entry
    Russell, Graeme, 1947– .
    First-time father : the essential guide for the new dad / Graeme Russell and
    Tony White

    2nd edition.
    Includes index.
    ISBN 978 192 1462030 (pbk).

    1. Father and child. 2. Fatherhood. 3. Parenting. 4. Work and family.

Edited by Catherine J Page
Editorial assistance from Patricia Cortese
Text designed and typeset in Stone Serif ITC by Meg Dunworth
Cover design by Creation Graphics
Cover photograph courtesy of Baby Björn AB
Internal photographs courtesy of Bradon, Melissa and Harper Grace French; Dean
Tregenza and Annette Jackson; Timothy and Rachel Kleu; Hayley French, especially
for her photographic skills; Kirstine Russell and Damian, Leo, Hugo and Otto Hadley;
Graeme Russell; Terence, Steen and Kane Ledger; Benjamin, Tobias and Elliot Russell.
Illustrations by Roy Bisson
Printed by Griffin Press

Notes   The 'Authors' notes' section at the back of this book contains useful
additional information and references to quoted material in the text. Each
reference is linked to the text by its relevant page number and an identifying
line entry.

Other Finch titles can be viewed at www.finch.com.au

Contents

Introduction

The research shows that what you do as a father matters: to your child, to your partner, and to you. Getting involved from the very beginning provides you with countless opportunities to enrich your journey as a father; this can benefit you, your child, your family, and even your workplace! Such has been the experience of many of the fathers we have worked with.

Fathers today are seeking a range of different options to help them be the kind of fathers *they* want to be. While most aim to develop a strong and enduring relationship with their children, some find it important to be actively involved in day-to-day care and decision-making concerning their children. This can mean sharing the parenting and paid work equally with their partner, taking extended leave from paid work to be the primary caregiver for a period of time, or reducing their hours of work (e.g. to work part-time) to be highly involved in caring for their child.

Today, more men and women want a successful career as well as a satisfying family life, and many parents with young children are both in the paid workforce. More couples are seeking to base their relationships on equality, in terms of paid work and in caring for their children. Society's changing expectations, as well as new workplace policies reflecting these changes, are giving couples more options to support their aspirations.

The research and our experience both show that approaching fatherhood with the following five things in mind can be very beneficial:

✶ **What is best for my child?** How do I decide what I want for my child? What are his needs, and how can I make sure I meet these? (This might not always be obvious!)

★ **How can I connect with my newborn, and stay connected with her as she grows?** What are my opportunities to be actively involved, to be part of my child's life from the beginning, to share the joys and challenges as she grows – to be a positive influence in her life? How can I build a strong relationship with my child?

★ **What about my partner: how can we work together? How can we work as a team?** The research evidence shows the value of a strong relationship with your partner and the benefits that result for your child from working as a parenting 'team' (also called co-parenting).

★ **How can I include my child in my life?** Are there benefits in integrating the needs of my child into all aspects of my life? What strategies can help me balance my work with my new family responsibilities?

★ **What impact do fathers have, and how important are they?** Will I be included in all aspects of the pregnancy, birth and beyond? Am I important from the beginning? Do I only matter when my child is older and needs discipline or wants to play sport?

The good news is that this book taps a substantial body of evidence that can help you plan a rewarding and effective fatherhood journey.

What a journey fatherhood is! Fatherhood changes our lives in ways that few of us are able to anticipate. Like any journey, it will at times be exhilarating and rewarding, and at other times challenging and uncertain, with difficult decisions to make. Rewards come from being an important part of your child's own journey and from sharing the experience with your partner – being in the front seat to share the pleasures, the challenges and the responsibilities. Importantly, you need to be in the front seat because fathers matter to children! Fathers make a difference to the lives of children, and children make a difference to their father's lives as well.

Children benefit from parents working together from the beginning. To be part of this team it is critical for you to feel valued as a father and to know that you are important to your child.

In the many years that we have worked with new parents, we have not met a single father who did not want the best for his child. A common challenge for fathers though is to turn this motivation into action – to be the kind of dads they want to be. In our work, as in this book, we have attempted to provide support and options that enable fathers to be involved and share with their partners the fun and responsibilities that go with being a parent.

The following poem was developed as part of a program to support first-time dads. It identifies the commitment of many first-time fathers – a commitment often not stated but from our

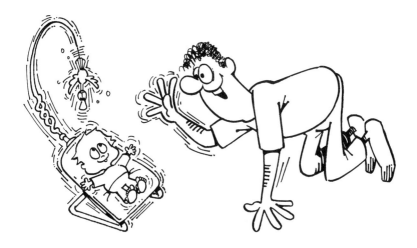

experience readily accepted when prospective dads realise just how important they are to their child.

I'm a dad
I want to be involved from the start
knowing I'm important to my child;

I'll share the sleepless nights and walk the floor
knowing I'm important to my child;

I'll change nappies, hold gently
and talk to my baby
knowing I'm important to my child;

I'll be there for my baby
knowing I'm important to my child;

I will grow as a person and share my feelings,
my dreams and my fears
knowing I'm important to my child;

I will share the joys
and difficulties
of parenting with my partner
knowing we are both important to our child.

What will you find in this book?

This book has been written primarily with the new father in mind. Importantly though, we discuss a diversity of fatherhood perspectives – in terms of age, family context, aspirations and personal resources. We focus on several key themes to give you a more rewarding experience as a reader. These are to:

Celebrate   Being a father is something to celebrate and value as part of your life.

Affirm   We emphasise your importance as a father to your child, to your family and to the broader community.

Reflect   Reading this book provides you with the opportunity to reflect on your role as a father – to take the time to consider what is important to you and what you want for your child. It also provides you with the opportunity to reflect on your relationship with your partner and the importance of working together throughout your child's life.

Share   The book provides an opportunity for you to share your journey with a broad range of other fathers.

Learn   Included in the book is important information about your child, from conception to the early months of life, and ideas to support your involvement from the very beginning.

We have structured the chapters around your journey as a new father.

Chapter 1   focuses on what new fathers say they want and on what is important in the initial stages of planning for your journey. We look at what is essential for your child, your relationship and you.

Chapter 2   takes a step back to consider what the latest research tells us about fathers and the influences they have.

Chapter 3   covers the major life changes experienced by fathers: an increased sense of responsibility, different sleep patterns and daily habits, a change in financial situation, adjusted work commitments and, possibly, a change in the nature of your relationship with your partner.

Chapter 4 describes the pregnancy journey. It covers all you need to know about what happens during pregnancy: the different stages (first, second and third trimesters), what is happening to the baby, what is happening to your partner, what you can do to be involved and to support your partner, what you need to do for your baby and what to expect from childbirth education classes.

Chapter 5 is about labour and the birth. The key issues covered are: fathers' experiences of labour and the birth, what is happening at each stage, how to become part of the team and how to celebrate the arrival of your baby.

Chapter 6 focuses on coming home and the vital first six weeks. Some of the issues we cover in this chapter are: fathers' feelings and responses to coming home with a baby, the type of involvement that is possible for fathers, getting to know your baby and responding to her needs, and getting it together as a team.

Chapter 7 is about what a baby needs. This is written from the perspective of a baby – you will certainly notice the different voice! Here, we cover crying, sleeping, feeding, changing and bathing baby – all you need to know to respond to the needs of your baby.

Chapter 8 is about connecting as a dad. This chapter covers the importance of father–child attachment – the fundamental relationship you will have with your child – as well as what you can do to stay connected.

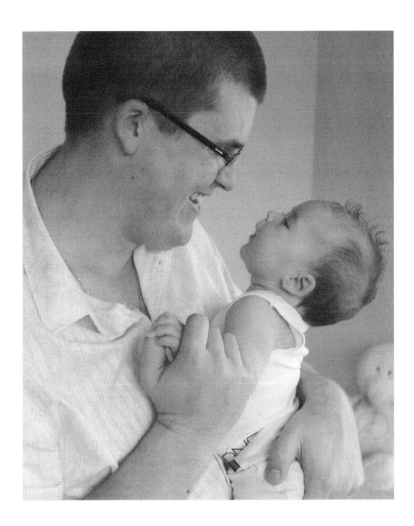

Chapter 9 is about balancing work and family life. Most fathers experience some difficulties in navigating their commitment to their job and the demands of having a new baby. This chapter provides you with some strategies for making this work better for you.

In these chapters we answer many of the questions you will have and provide ideas and alternatives about how you might approach being a dad. The ideas we present come from three main sources:

1 the experiences of other fathers – fathers who we have worked with, talked to and listened to

2 the growing body of research on fathers and the influence they have on their children (we give you the latest evidence on the importance of fathers)

3 our own personal experience as men and fathers (and from our debate and discussion with each other!). We are both fathers and grandfathers, and we have been conducting research and providing services for fathers and families for a combined total of over 70 years!

So, let the journey begin.

Note: In the interests of equity, we use 'she' and 'he' in alternating chapters when talking about non-specific babies.

1 New questions for new fathers

Very few of us cross the bridge into fatherhood with a clear view of what it will be like. And while there will be some common ground, there will also be differences in how each of us experiences this life stage. Even if we were to read the same books and attend the same parent education classes, our fatherhood feelings and experiences could still be surprisingly different. We all start from different points and encounter different challenges along the way. What we see and experience, who travels with us, what our babies are like – all of these things contribute to the diversity of being a dad.

Having questions and concerns as a father is common. This is because we want to be good fathers, and because we want the very best for our children. We develop our ideas about being a father from a range of sources, including our own experiences as a child, what we have seen and what we have read. Some of us use our own father as a guide to our new role:

> 'I want to be like my dad – he was always there when I needed him and he was so patient.'

> 'My father was never around – he spent a lot of time at work. I want to be there for my children.'

Others may base their ideas on a range of men they have observed or read about; and still others might not even have thought about it:

> 'I kind of stumbled into fatherhood – I knew that I should and would be a good father, but I didn't know what that meant.'

There is no single pathway to being an effective or good dad. What we do as a father is influenced by our experiences and our current circumstances. How you experience fatherhood is influenced by how you prepare for the journey and how you are involved – from pregnancy onwards. And without a doubt, you will be involved in some way or another!

This is what a group of six fathers said when we asked them what they thought about soon becoming dads. This provides you with an opportunity to reflect on your own ideas by listening in on the experiences of other fathers.

What fathers say

'Karen and I had been together about a year. We spent the last two months planning an overseas holiday – every day – three months in Asia, six months in South America and at least twelve months in Europe. We had worked out budgets and work opportunities and had purchased open tickets so we could travel as long as we wanted. Then three weeks before we were to leave she told me we were going to have a baby. The first thing I said to her was "Does it need a passport?" Karen cried both with joy and with disappointment. I was so focused on our trip that I said I'd check *Lonely Planet* to see what it said about pregnant travellers. Let me tell you, *Lonely Planet* didn't cover travelling while pregnant. We cancelled our trip and I tried hard to make out I was happy. She became a bit suspicious when I suggested that the baby should be called "Asia". I'd be lying if I said that I didn't resent the "thing" that was stopping me from seeing the world. I loved Karen but I had little interest in the pregnancy. I didn't talk about it and I avoided all Karen's appointments with the doctor. It wasn't until the labour that I really got involved. At first it was concern about Karen. Then I saw our baby born and it all changed. Our son looked like ET but something happened to me that I can't explain. I fell in love again. Stuff the trip, I had something better – a son.'

Gerard, 27

How we react to becoming a dad will vary and be affected by our life experiences and current circumstances. How we deal with our reactions is important.

'We're going to have a baby. How do I feel? What are my thoughts – what am I looking forward to? Do I have any concerns? I'm not sure. The first person I rang was my father. I don't know why. I'm not particularly close to him and I can't say that he has been the best dad in the world. He was around, but not what you would call engaged. Perhaps I felt a need to share it with him first because I knew how enthusiastic he was about being a grandfather. If I wanted to be cynical, I could say it was because he wanted to make up for what he thinks he missed out on with us – maybe it's guilt. He is retired now so he does have more time. This is his first grandchild, so I figured he should be excited. And yes, he was. I think he was more excited than I was. We didn't talk for very long. We didn't have a heart to heart, nor did he give me any advice. After saying it was great and that he couldn't wait, he asked the standard questions. When is the baby due? How is Amanda? Is she well? Funny now that I think about it, he didn't ask me how I felt. Not many people do; most focus on the baby and Amanda.'

Blake, 32

Wouldn't it be wonderful if people did take the trouble to ask dads how they feel at all stages of the journey. This is part of being included – and indeed valued.

'Those kinds of comments didn't bother me – I am what some people call a "mature father". Sure, I am a bit older than most. On the other hand, I have had a lot more time to think, plan and to fantasise. I am ready. To me this is the big game, the main match of life – the big trip. I want to be a dad, I want to be involved, to be there, to see and experience everything.'

John, 48

Wanting to be involved from the beginning is a great start to John's journey.

'I have some of those feelings as well. Most people focus on Louise and the baby. I was very excited when the test was positive. We knew, though, that the test was just the confirmation. Louise is very regular and we had been trying for some time. We both wanted to have children. Both my sisters have children and I was feeling a little left out. I can't wait. It is going to be fantastic to have a child around, to have fun with, to be a friend. I expect that it will slow me down a little too, but then I probably need that. I tend to focus too much on my work and myself. This should put a bit more balance in my life.'

Harvey, 24

'Balance in your life? From what I hear from my mates at work who have had children, it puts a lot more pressure on your life. They were great when they found out we were having a baby. They congratulated me, and made a few jokes, but I thought they were genuinely interested. It has opened up a new conversation with them. I think I am beginning to understand some of the challenges they experience. I hadn't really thought about it until the reality of Joan being pregnant hit me. Don't get me wrong, I want to have children too. It will mean that we will be a family – being a couple was great, but being a family will be even better. I'm looking forward to being a father. But there is the added responsibility – and the costs (my mates keep reminding me of this). I expect there to be added demands as well. I feel some uncertainty about this, maybe even a little anxious as I am not 100 per cent clear about what to expect.'

Byron, 31

'There will be added demands and responsibilities, but I look on this as a positive thing – it's an opportunity. It will be a challenge, but what comes with it I expect to be fully worth it. As I see it, things have changed and fathers have more options today. Look at my family situation. Both Sharon and I have full-time jobs, and both of us expect to work after we have our baby. This is very different from the families we both grew up in where our mums stayed at home and our dads went to work. Our dads were both traditional breadwinners, but they also took their fathering responsibilities very seriously. They provided us with security and they were loving. But to me now – well the way I am looking at being a dad – they missed out on a lot too. I see myself as having more options than my father – he wasn't at the birth of any of his children, and from what I hear from other fathers, this is an absolute high –

something not to be missed. It is more accepted today for fathers to be involved in everything. There is more support for this too. Indeed, there is some expectation that fathers will be involved. I know Sharon wants this – she sees it as an equity issue just as she wants to pursue her career. Maybe it is an equity issue for me as well – that I have equal time as a parent. Other things have changed as well at work. I can get one week's paid paternity leave from my employer. I will definitely be taking this. My workplace also has the option of part-time work. This is something I might consider as well.'

Andrew, 35

Following up on the comments of Andrew above, the research shows that many more fathers today are highly involved in parenting. They are what we might call 'active' dads – dads who take responsibility for the day-to-day care of their children (sometimes sharing this with their partners while they both have paid jobs), dads who give equal priority to parenting and their work. Overall they are dads who actively seek to connect with their children and to influence their children's development from the very beginning.

We have seen positive changes in the way the staff of services designed to support parents and the general community view the role of fathers. While there are still challenges, there are now many advocates attempting to change attitudes so that dads are valued, included and supported at *all* stages of their journey. Your contribution to this change involves believing that you are important and getting involved from the very beginning.

And things keep changing in the workplace too. Andrew will find that he has the right to request flexibility when his child is under school age or if he has a child under 18 with a disability. There is more on this new development in Chapter 9 (p. 200).

The pathways to fatherhood have been different for our six dads but they are all starting a journey that will provide opportunities for them to make a difference in the lives of their children.

Our aim is to enable you to explore these opportunities and to provide you with encouragement and support in your exciting new journey as a dad. As a result of reading this book, we hope that:

★ You will be energised and inspired – and even more enthusiastic about being a father. *Celebrate* being a father and enjoy the experience! Take your time and savour every moment.

★ You will know that fathers are important – that *fathers matter* and that they make a significant contribution to their children – and that *you can make a difference* to your child's journey in life. You will see this in your child's eyes, in your child's recognition of you and in the hugs you will share.

★ You understand and act on the five steps outlined in this chapter for enhancing your experience as a father. These are the major challenges and opportunities for you as a father. Being a father is like all of our journeys in life – they all have a balance of pleasure and pain.

The previous comments from the six fathers help to clarify what kinds of things fathers start out seeking – what they want as fathers, what is going through their minds and what are they wondering about.

Five steps in the pathway to effective fatherhood

1. Focus on what is best for your child

What you need to do first is answer two questions: 'What do I want for my child?' and 'What does my child need?' Then, focus on how you can achieve what you want for your child and how you can satisfy her needs.

★ **What do you want for your child?** What are your aspirations? How would you like your child to turn out? Most mothers and fathers want the same things: a happy, healthy and secure child who has roots (a sense of identity and values) and wings (a sense of independence).

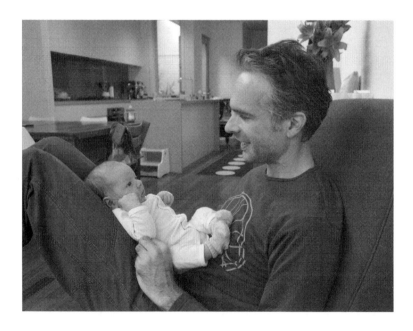

What can you do?

Start your own parenting diary or dialogue. Agree on a time with your partner to have a discussion about what you each want for your child. Perhaps you could write a summary of this and review it regularly to check on how you are doing or to revise your aspirations.

★ **What does your child need?** In the early weeks and months, we may tend to focus more on a child's physical needs, such as food, sleep and physical comfort. However, they have equally important social and psychological needs, such as being responded to, loved and cuddled. Most fathers want to know what makes their children grow, what makes them happy, what makes them safe, what children should be doing at various stages (e.g. when most babies begin to smile, how much weight they tend to put on in the first month), and what the danger signs are, so you know when to seek medical assistance. From the research (see Chapter 2), we know that fathers can become competent and skilled caregivers, sensitive to their new baby's cues and providing the comfort a baby needs. Once it was believed that only mothers were capable of this. Like most other tasks in life, the effective care of a baby requires you to be committed and motivated (you have to want to do it!), have the necessary knowledge and skills, have support, and engage in regular practice to achieve mastery!

'At first it all seemed overwhelming but we had been advised to stick to the basics and we would learn from cues given by our baby. We were told this was "working with the baby". We didn't always guess right but we got better at it.'

This book provides you with the necessary information to enable you to understand your baby's needs from the beginning of pregnancy to the early months of their lives. We also present options that will help you to respond in ways that best meet your child's needs.

What can you do?

Read this book. You may also build on your knowledge by seeking out additional information on the needs of children. For example, check out your local library or bookshop, or one of the websites listed at the end of this book. Or you could have a look at one of the many books that your partner has no doubt bought. You might also consider having a chat to other fathers, asking your own parents, or reflecting upon your own life – what really mattered to you when you were growing up? Another important way of gaining information is to attend appointments with your partner and to ask questions of the service providers – your doctor, midwife and child and family nurse.

2. Connect with your child

Some of the questions to consider are:

⋆ What are my options as a father?

⋆ What is it that a parent does that makes a difference to children?

⋆ Are mothers and fathers both important?

As was noted by Andrew above, fathers have more options today than they did in previous generations. More fathers today want to be involved in the day-to-day care of their children, more want to actively engage in their children's lives and more want to ensure that they make a difference to their children's development.

The clear message from the research is that fathers matter and that mothers and fathers are both very important to their children.

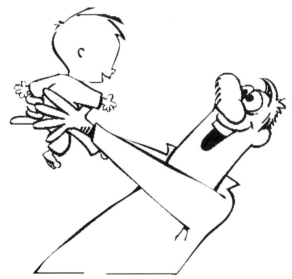

'Do dads matter? Of course my dad matters! What a silly question! I love my dad, I love the games we play, I love the way he smiles at me (he thinks I'm smiling back – but I'm not that advanced yet) and the faces he pulls. He certainly looks proud of me. He cares for me, he rocks me to sleep and he talks funny to me. We really have fun together. He is impatient for me to wake up when he comes home from work. He bathes me – he has bigger hands than Mum. I can tell he loves me.'
Emily, 4 months

In children's eyes, fathers have always mattered. The majority of children seek to know, understand and have acceptance from their fathers – they seek affection from and are comforted by their fathers. They want to know their fathers and have a good relationship with them. And fathers want this too!

This might seem obvious. Yet fathers are often seen as being the secondary parent, the support person or mother's helper. Sometimes it is assumed that parenting comes naturally to mothers and that all women make good mothers – they are the experts – and that mothers have the major influence over children. The reality is quite different from this. Research shows that babies become attached to both fathers and mothers – it depends on the parent responding sensitively and lovingly to their needs and providing enjoyable and playful stimulation. These are all things that both dads and mums can do.

At the most fundamental and critical level, your impact will depend very much on the nature of the relationship you develop with your child and, particularly, on how you stay connected – both in terms of your availability to your child and the ways in which you interact with your child.

What can you do?

Write a summary of the kind of dad you want to be and share this with your partner or with a friend who is already a father. Talk to your own father about your ideas too. Consider the full range of possibilities.

For some fathers in previous generations, fatherhood was reasonably straightforward. They had a job, they provided for their families, they were involved in disciplining (for some children it was 'wait until your father gets home!') and in most of the major decisions (e.g. which school, which sport). The day-to-day care, however, was usually looked after by mothers. In recent times researchers have spent some effort trying to define and measure fathers' involvement, and it now looks much more expansive and complex.

Some of the options you might consider are:

- Have a sense of perspective as a father by keeping in mind the need for children to have both roots (security) and wings (independence).
- Be open, curious and ready to learn about being a father.
- Be ready to experience the feelings and joys of being a parent: celebrate.
- Be actively engaged and connected with your child.
- Develop skills to resolve tensions and differences with your partner.
- Reduce your hours at work.
- Develop strategies to achieve harmony between your work and family responsibilities.
- Take some responsibility for caregiving tasks – from the beginning.

And at all times remember – *you are important to your child*.

3. Be a team: it takes two (and more!)

As we have already mentioned, being a parent is a challenging responsibility, and there is a lot to do. At times you might find yourself stretched to the limit, both psychologically (e.g. not being able to figure out why your baby won't sleep) and physically (e.g. not having enough sleep). It is extremely difficult for one person to be fully, or even mainly, responsible for all the needs of a child. Many people find that things work out better if they adopt a team approach, in every aspect of parenting.

Most of us have belonged to a team at some time – at work or in sport. We have all heard about the benefits of 'working as a team'. It is often said in sport that 'a good team will beat a team of good individuals'. Working as a 'parenting team' will benefit you, your child and your relationship with your partner.

Effective teams rarely just happen. You need:

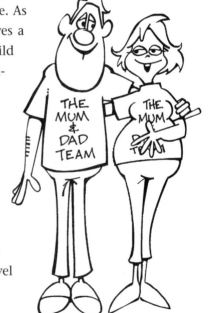

* **A shared vision** – agreement on what you want to achieve. As parents this often involves a happy and healthy child who grows into a well-adjusted adult.

* **Common goals** – what you want to achieve during each stage or leg of the journey. Some of these you can plan at the beginning but many you will develop as you travel on your journey.

* **Consistency** – this will involve agreement on parenting styles and approaches to day-to-day childrearing (e.g. sleep patterns, feeding).

* **Good communication** – a critical part of effective teamwork. How you communicate was important from the start of your relationship and will be tested as you travel together as parents.

Clearly, the founding members of this team are the mother and father. In a strong partnership, each party will exercise leadership at various times, and each is prepared to take on different roles. Being sensitive to and caring for the needs of your partner is also a key part of the teamwork approach (e.g. the need for both of you to have personal time). You will also find that at times you need others, such as doctors, nurses, grandparents or neighbours, to join your team.

What can you do?

* Have a discussion with your partner about what your partnership will be like and who the critical members of your team will be at various times – you will need all the help you can get.
* Have clear goals about what you are trying to achieve in terms of your child's development.
* Agree on how these goals can be achieved and what your roles will be. Many couples find it best if they are not too rigid about who does what – it is better to combine specialisation with multiskilling.
* Have a discussion about fairness and equity in your relationship and consider how each of you will

balance paid work, caring for your child and having time for yourself. Try to avoid arguments about what you think male and female roles are.

- Consider what your processes will be. How will you communicate (e.g. consider when you will have regular discussions – perhaps each weekend; it makes good sense to plan for these), problem solve (e.g. about why your baby is not as contented as you expected or would like) and resolve conflicts (e.g. about different styles of putting your baby to sleep)?

- Place a high priority on your relationship and look for ways to keep it alive. Consider how to develop and demonstrate trust and openness, recognition and support. How can you get on well together and share a sense of belonging; how can you maintain and show your importance in each other's lives.

- Be aware of outside factors that may affect your team. Some fathers report difficulties with the level of involvement of grandparents – for example, they may be all too willing to give advice, and may tend to take over when they are around. You might also find that pressures at work, or advice your partner receives from an early childhood nurse, might challenge how you work as a team. Even though these external factors might be out of your control, it is important to recognise them and their potential impact. And you *can* control your response to them.

4. Strengthen your relationship with your partner

Your relationship with your partner can come under stress during your transition to parenthood. This is a huge life change and the focus is on the baby – as it should be. The changes in your life – sleep deprivation, feelings of being overwhelmed, possible conflicts between work and home, lack of time for intimacy – can impact on the quality of your relationship with your partner. But it is important to remember that your relationship with your partner affects your child's development. Don't neglect the things that made your relationship strong – communication, patience, understanding, and of course love and respect for your partner. We have made recommendations to strengthen your relationship throughout the book, and the important points are:

★ Address any conflict in your relationship as soon as it arises – don't let it 'fester'.

★ Build a pattern of togetherness – share common activities and laughter, e.g. go to the movies, go for a walk together.

★ Explore sexual love and intimacy with your partner. Touching, holding and kissing based on tenderness make a difference!

★ Avoid criticising or blaming your partner. Try to make at least five positive communications for every negative one. Admire your partner and give genuine praise, e.g. 'You were really funny tonight, I love your sense of humour', 'I love watching you play with Emily'.

★ Accept 100 per cent responsibility for 50 per cent of your relationship.

★ Avoid violence of any kind – it can have serious long-term impacts on your baby.

★ Remember that you need time alone with your baby, personal time for you, time as a couple with the baby, and time as a couple without the baby – and your partner needs the same.

5. Include your child in your life

In the third chapter of this book we focus on the challenges most fathers experience in including a child in their lives. This is not

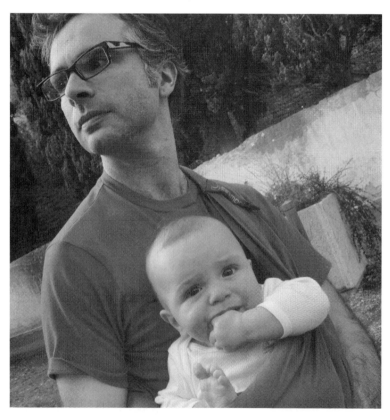

something that happens briefly and goes away; it is a long-term issue. In the initial stages it has more to do with adjusting to the day-to-day demands of a baby (e.g. most of us find our sleep patterns have to change). Another key issue is how to include your child in your broader life – work and leisure.

We hear a lot about work/life balance these days. For many of us, life has become very hectic and work demands have increased. Having a child adds a new dimension and for some provides extra challenges in terms of the use of time, and in terms of deciding on life priorities, especially in relation to the competing demands of work and family life. The big challenge here is how to include and integrate another person into your life. At some stages this will become an issue for you as the financial provider (e.g. if you have only one income for a period of time) and at others it will revolve around making adjustments to your work (e.g. if you want to be home earlier) and to your career aspirations (e.g. to delay your career advancement for a period of time) to enable you to give priority to your family, and especially to your child. This might also mean challenging commonly accepted attitudes and behaviours at your workplace. These issues are discussed in Chapter 9.

What can you do?

Have a discussion with your partner about what you see as your major strengths and challenges in terms of adjusting to life with a child. Talk to another father to gain a reality check on your expectations.

Consider developing a financial plan and a longer term strategy for both your own and your partner's involvement in paid work.

Summary

★ Everyone's thoughts about what fatherhood will be like are different.
★ Fathers do matter and do make a difference to their children's lives.
★ Focusing on what you want for your child, and her needs, is important; and it is equally important to connect with your child as a dad.
★ Caring for a child is a team effort, with the mother and father leading the team in partnership.
★ Fully including your child in your life is a challenge, but it is necessary if you want to raise a happy, independent child.

2 The latest research on fathering

In this chapter we take a step back and consider what the research tells us about fathering (what you actually do), in terms of both what influences fathers have and how the process of fathers influencing their children actually occurs. It is no surprise that what mothers and fathers do, both individually and together, has a significant impact on the wellbeing of their children, on their partners and on themselves – although the impact that being a father has on fathers is something that is often overlooked. What does come as a surprise to us is the continuing quest by researchers to demonstrate that fathers matter and that they have a unique or essential contribution to a child's development (e.g. one that is linked to masculinity).

Mothers, fathers and children know that fathers are important, and research continues to confirm this. It is true that, on average, fathers have more choices or options than mothers in terms of how involved they are. Fathers are more likely to be in the paid workforce, and they are also less likely than mothers to have cared for children in the past (e.g. their younger siblings or as paid babysitters).

Fundamentally, parenting is about what children need – not about the gender of the caregiver – and your child needs you to be actively involved in his life. Children actively seek a quality relationship with their fathers. Your child will also model or adopt different things from you and from their mother, as much as anything else because you are different people!

What do children need from their fathers?

What you do with your children is influenced by many factors – your upbringing, your relationship with your own father, your partner's expectations, your level of motivation, and so on. This means that fathering is expressed in a diversity of ways, and involves a range of behaviours and responsibilities. These can include:

1 **Being positively engaged with your child.** This involves taking the initiative and getting involved with your child in a highly active way, such as physical play with toys or simply lying on the floor with your baby, singing and talking to him; taking responsibility for the daily care of your child (e.g. while your partner goes to the gym or goes out with friends); or sharing in caregiving tasks such as bathing and changing nappies. These are all activities that will increase your salience to your child. He will come to anticipate and seek this type of involvement from you.

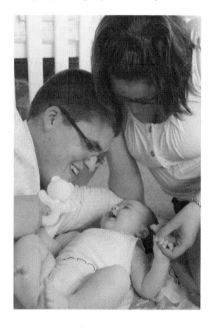

2 **Being warm and responsive towards your child.** This involves being attentive and responsive to your child's needs, e.g. cuddling him and being affectionate (simply

sitting with him and having a quiet moment), soothing and settling him when he is crying (and you can't figure out what the problem is!), or rocking him to sleep.

3   **Monitoring your baby and making decisions about his needs.** This includes monitoring his physical health and wellbeing (e.g. is he having enough sleep, do we need to review the routines we have established to help him self-settle) and sharing in decision-making about changing his sleep and feeding patterns.

4   **Indirect care.** Activities done for your child, but not with him, e.g. buying toys or clothes, increasing your knowledge about child development, monitoring the latest evidence about the needs of babies, going to a workshop for fathers etc.

'I'm not sure I had given much thought to what fathering would look like, or to the kind of father I would be. I took four weeks off work when Grace was five weeks old. It soon became clear to me that all options were open to me. I got into fathering full pelt; I became a greater talker, listener and singer. I was also highly competitive about getting the first smile from Grace. I was into bathing, cuddling her when she was upset and putting her to sleep. I also had the chance to read more about early development and found some great websites. Soon Sally and I were constantly sharing experiences and debating and discussing feeding and sleeping patterns. Our sex life also started to get back on track. And, best of all, I found that I had got into tune with Grace; I felt confident in being able to read her signals and anticipate her needs.'

Harry, 31

Fathers are competent caregivers

The latest research affirms Harry's experience, telling us that fathers have the capabilities to be sensitive, nurturing and attentive to their newborns. They are competent carers, responding to the uniqueness of their own newborn and adjusting their speech patterns when interacting with their infants. Fathers are just as sensitive as mothers to their child's needs and signals throughout the first year of life. This is an important finding, because earlier research focused only on mothers; it was commonly believed that fathers were not as competent as mothers in caring for their newborn babies. This finding opens up many more opportunities for you as a father. A good first step is to regularly spend some time alone with your newborn, so that you can develop your own relationship with him.

Being warm and caring towards your child makes the biggest difference

While the process of influence for fathers is the same as for mothers, research consistently shows that fathers' behaviours influence children's outcomes independently of mothers' behaviours. For both parents, warmth, nurturance and closeness are associated with more positive outcomes for children.

Fathers who are positively engaged in child-focused activities, who are consistently warm and accepting of their children, and who are responsive to their child's needs and signals (e.g. by actively engaging in play or comforting a baby to help settle him to sleep), have the greatest impact on the long-term wellbeing of their children. This impact has been found consistently at all

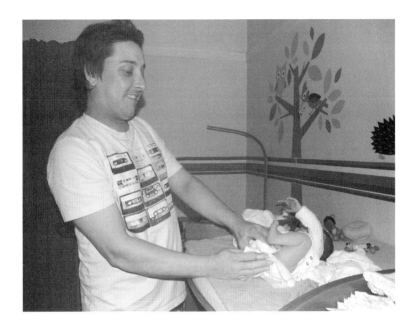

stages of a child's development, and research has now examined some of the longer-term effects of fathering on children.

For example, in one of the most widely cited studies, active involvement by a father in the pre-school years resulted in lower levels of delinquency in teenage sons, and a father's interest in his child's education was associated with adult daughters' levels of educational achievement. In a recent Australian study, fathers with high levels of warmth and self-efficacy (that is, fathers who felt they had the knowledge or skills to fulfil the role of being a good parent and were confident in what they did as a father – like Harry above) were found to have children who got on better with their friends and had more advanced language, literacy and mathematical skills. The actual amount of time fathers spent with their children was not related to child outcomes, meaning that what fathers do when they are there is more important.

'I went to a talk on fathers and the speaker mentioned the longer-term effects fathers can have on their children. It seemed a long way off to me and I wondered about the process and how I can have this much power given all the other possible influences on my child. It also made me reflect on my own upbringing. My dad wasn't all that involved and I've turned out OK. I also have a really good relationship with him now. I see him as a very important person in my life and I often go to him for advice. At the end of day, I did take away the positive point that as a dad I am an important person and that if I stick to the fundamentals – being available, getting involved and being warm and responsive, Alice will have a better start in life.'

Martin, 36.

Being warm and responsive to your baby as well as actively engaged in play and caring, and being available to your child, increases their motivation and opportunity to identify with you, feel close to you and model your behaviours.

In contrast with earlier notions of fatherhood and the influences fathers have on children, and especially on sons, the research tends to show that the quality of the father–child relationship is much more important in influencing children's wellbeing and how they turn out than are the characteristics of individual fathers, e.g. the strength of their 'masculinity'. Again, this emphasises the point that what you do with your child and how responsive you are to their needs is what matters most.

'One of the fathers at the antenatal class we went to kept asking questions about fathers and sons. It seemed that he had read something and that it had had a major impact on him. He was looking for affirmation that he was going to be especially important or critical to his son's development. We knew we were having a daughter and I kept thinking to myself that surely I was going to be a key part of my daughter's life.'

Joseph, 29

The quality of father–child interactions is also linked to the security of attachment between a child and her father. Secure parent–child attachment is accepted as a major determinant of positive outcomes for children. Most infants form attachments to fathers and mothers at about the same age (around seven to nine months); about two-thirds of all attachments to both fathers and mothers are rated as secure (that is, your child feels safe and comfortable with you); and there are no differences in the average levels of attachment security that infants have with their fathers and mothers. (If you'd like to learn more about attachment, see Chapter 8.)

'We had a very switched-on midwife who ran our antenatal class. She knew all the latest research and went out of her way to make sure the men were included, had the opportunity to ask questions and to talk about their concerns. It surprised me just how open the men were, I hadn't experienced this before. What I found particularly fascinating was the discussion we had about attachment. I had never thought of young babies as having this capacity; knowing who their parents are and having an emotional or security response to them. This helped give me a kick start as a father, to know that my child sees me as important. This is backed up be scientific evidence. It is not just my imagination!'

Grant, 41

Being an active father is good for fathers and mothers

Both fathers and mothers benefit from fathers being actively involved in parenting.

1   The involvement of fathers during pregnancy is positively related to the health of both fathers (particularly their psychological wellbeing – e.g. an increased sense of maturity and responsibility) and mothers (particularly their physical health).

2   More generally, fathers who are actively involved with their children have:
    ★ an increased sense of maturity and more patience (across all areas of their lives)
    ★ a more positive self-image, or higher levels of self-esteem
    ★ a partner with higher levels of psychological wellbeing and self-esteem, and more success in paid work
    ★ a better quality marital or couple relationship.

'No question, being a father has changed me as a person and it has changed my view of the world. I now place more value on the importance of ensuring children get the very best start in life that they can. I have also changed some of my behaviours and habits. It might be hard to believe, especially for my group of mates, but I now take fewer risks on the roads. I have also gone to my doctor to have a general health check-up. This is something I had never done before.'

Hans, 35

Having a high quality co-parenting relationship makes a difference

Research consistently shows that the quality of the relationship you have with your partner – who does what (in terms of childcare and housework), how much you support or undermine your partner, and the level of agreement you have on child-rearing practices – has an impact on your child's wellbeing. We now know that:

1 Fathers are more involved and adopt a more positive approach to parenting (e.g. they display more warmth to their child) when their partners are more supportive of them as fathers.

2 Fathers in happier co-parenting relationships spend more time on childcare.

3 Fathers with happier relationships with their partners adopt a more positive approach to parenting.

4 The support parents give to each other has a positive impact on their children's emotional wellbeing.

The nature of the relationship you have with your partner is something you really need to keep your eye on. Research conducted by John Gottman and his associates showed that in the first three years of a child's life, 67 per cent of parents experienced a decline in their relationship satisfaction, and this decline was associated with an increase in hostility. Critically, it was also found that in families with higher quality couple relationships, as indicated by the level of support, agreement and intimacy, the fathers were more involved with their children. Further, couples with lower quality relationships also had lower skills in reading their baby's emotional signals and were far less responsive to their baby – and as was indicated earlier, being responsive to a baby's signals is a strong predictor of positive outcomes for children.

The good news is that these researchers have developed a program to help parents negotiate the transition to parenthood by developing higher quality relationships.

Work and fatherhood

A common assumption is that workplace demands, a lack of workplace flexibility (particularly in terms of leave provisions), and men's strong identification with both paid work and career success are the major barriers to active involvement as a father, and especially involvement in caring for their young children.

Being the breadwinner or financial provider has been seen as both a major component of the contribution fathers make to the wellbeing of their families, and a major constraint on their active involvement in family life. Yet there has been surprisingly little research into the relationship between a father's involvement in his job and what he does as father, nor on the impact that the demands of his job have on child wellbeing.

With increased expectations that fathers be more involved and take greater responsibility for their children, as well as the trend for more mothers to be employed, the impact that paid work has on fathering and children has become a topic of greater interest.

Findings are generally consistent in showing that higher levels of workplace demands, or role overload, reduce the quality of father–child interactions. Fathers with high work demands are less accepting of their children, express more anger towards their children and are more emotionally withdrawn from family life. They can also be less capable of focusing on the needs of their child – something that we know makes a major difference to the wellbeing of children.

Recent US research findings also indicate that the level of work–life conflict experienced by fathers in dual-earner couples has increased over the past 30 years; it is now higher than that experienced by mothers in the same family situations. And recent Australian research shows that fathers with higher levels of negative work-to-family spillover (who feel that they are missing out at home or who find family time less enjoyable because of work) spend less time on childcare and are less supportive of their partners as parents. These fathers also report that they show lower levels of warmth towards their children.

These findings emphasise the importance of successfully integrating work and family responsibilities, especially for fathers of young children. Even if you have a demanding job, getting the balance right can enable you to develop high-quality relationships with your children (for more on this, see Chapter 9).

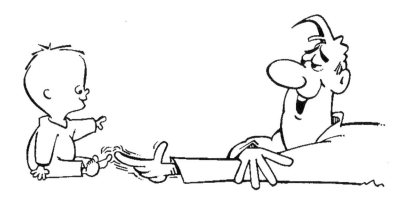

Summary

★ Research in the last 30 years shows that active involvement by fathers has a critical influence on the wellbeing of the whole family: children, mothers, fathers and the couple relationship.

★ Fatherhood is diverse and is expressed in many different ways. In many societies there is a continuing emphasis on a more involved model of fatherhood that encompasses both paid work and family caregiving, and a family pattern that involves both parents being in the paid workforce.

★ We need to shift our thinking to better understand the complex interactions between paid work and fatherhood, to explore ways in which workplace policies and practices restrict or enable active involvement, and how work and family life both conflict with and enhance each other. Paid work and fathering both have a role to play in facilitating wellbeing: of fathers, of the broader family system and of the community.

★ The research also strongly supports the importance of your relationship with your partner and its impact on outcomes for your child.

3 Life changes

There is one certainty for all new parents – your lives change when your babies arrive. How much change you each experience will depend on the nature of your baby (all babies differ), your current lifestyle, the quality of the relationship you currently have with your partner, your own resources/resilience, your coping strategies and your expectations, as well as the availability of other team members, such as grandparents. Having some idea about what to expect is usually helpful in adjusting to the actual event that changes all our lives – in this case, the introduction of a child.

Both mothers and fathers report similar challenges in the transition to parenthood. The six most critical changes are:

* **The additional responsibility of caring for your baby** – being constantly alert and always considering the needs of the baby.

* **The amount of time you have for yourself.** Most fathers find they have to make adjustments to their time commitments outside the home, such as the amount of time they spend on personal leisure and being with their friends.

* **Your sleep and daily habits** – such as the adjustment you might need to make to the quiet time you might have spent reading the paper in the morning, having a long shower or relaxing when you came home from work.

★ **Your financial situation.** Most couples experience a reduction in income and at the same time an increased demand for spending to look after the needs of their baby. This can be a significant challenge!

★ **Your commitment to paid work.** Many fathers find that their energy levels are lower, they are not able to concentrate as well at work and, of course, there are increased demands on their time. Research shows that over 50 per cent of fathers make some adjustment to their work patterns as a result of having a child (e.g. they may change jobs to one that is less demanding, come home earlier on some days of the week, or not seek a promotion for a period of time).

★ **Your relationship with your partner.** Having a baby can have a significant impact on the time you are able to spend together, how you communicate with each other and the extent of love and intimacy you share.

What can you do?

Before reading the next section, take the time to imagine that your baby has come home with you and your partner. Ask yourself how your life will change. Write down your responses in your parenting diary or on a piece of paper.

Now, let's take a trip to the future in company with a group of parents talking about their experiences when their first child was twelve months old. (Note: It is not an easy task to get a group of parents together at a mutually convenient time!)

Increased responsibility

'When I thought about being a dad I got worried. I didn't know anything about babies. They seemed so fragile and helpless. It seemed scary to think our baby would be completely dependent on us. I didn't have a clue about what to expect. I wanted to be involved from the start but I didn't know if I would be doing the right thing. How would I know if the baby was sick? I talked to my partner and discovered she felt the same. I thought women knew all this baby stuff. She told me she probably knew less than me. Our baby is doing very well and has survived in our house!'

Adam, 37

'I could not believe the level of commitment needed. We had always had pets, and I thought they needed a lot of attention – and that we sometimes paid them too much attention. But, having a baby tops it all off. There is no comparison. You have to constantly think about your baby – and worry, is she alright? Is she still alive? They are so dependent on you. It is a huge responsibility.'

Jacob, 29

'I agree. I had trouble recognising this initially. I just wasn't prepared for the enormity of the task. I had to move over and make some space in my thinking and about what was really important in life. Mind you, it feels good to have someone dependent on you like this and to provide the care for them. The responsibility was constant; it wasn't something – and still isn't – that you could farm out, or pay someone else to do.'

Brad, 29

> 'Yes, it's a bit like driving a car at night in a fog with all of your family there with you. You might be tired, but you have to stay alert, watching for danger signs, being constantly vigilant and focusing on the responsibility you have to get everyone home safely.'
>
> Hugh, 35

The thought of a small, helpless baby being totally dependent on you can indeed be scary – for men and for women. Contrary to popular belief, women do not come with built-in knowledge and skills to care for a baby. Unless they have previous experience in caring for infants, they have to learn – just like you. This is a good reason for you to be around during the first week or so when you bring your baby home. As we outline in Chapter 6, most couples experience major challenges at this time, and for some men it is a surprise that their partner doesn't know much more than they do. In Chapter 6 we also discuss the experiences of other fathers and provide you with some suggestions to help you enjoy these early days with your new family.

Loss of time for you and your partner

> 'Time? What is time? I don't have any to myself now.'
>
> William, 34

> 'Yes, but it's a good time, don't you think? I can't wait to get home every afternoon. It is my special time with my daughter, and on weekends. Every Sunday morning I take

her out somewhere (she now sleeps in the afternoons). This is probably the best thing I did at the beginning. I insisted on having my special time with her – alone with her, just Annabelle and me. It also meant that I didn't have too many heavy Saturday nights anymore. So, it's been a good thing for my health as well.'

Darren, 32

'The thing that struck me was that I found I didn't have any time to myself. Before our baby came along I was doing an hour's exercise every day and was playing soccer one night a week. Initially I gave all that up – I just couldn't find time to do it. But then I found I was putting on weight and getting a bit grumpy – I need time to myself. Louise was also very active before the birth and she was missing out too. I'm not sure how it happened, but we struck up a conversation one night after dinner about how our lives had changed and we both said that we missed the time for ourselves. We then came up with a strategy, a roster – or you might say a routine – to get exercise and personal time back into our lives. It took a bit of organisation and a bit of persistence to keep it going, but we each now do at least three hours' exercise each week. I have gone back to soccer (they were missing my curve balls) and Louise has a regular night out with her friends – not every week, usually more like once every three weeks.'

James, 38

Fathers report that along with time spent with their partner, one of the biggest changes they experience when they have children is the loss of time for themselves. As we outline in Chapter 9, there are good reasons for you to maintain focus on your personal wellbeing and taking care of yourself. You are important to your child – and having you around and healthy, with the energy to interact with her, is critical to her development.

Changed sleep and daily habits

'Sleep has always been important to me. Even though Carol and I had a few late nights before Sam was born, we knew that at some stage we could crash and catch up on our sleep. I remember talking to my mum before the birth and telling her I wanted a baby who sleeps most of the day and all through the night. She just looked at me, smiled and said, "Good luck, dear". In the sleep department I didn't get the one I wanted. Both Carol and I found the lack of sleep hard to take, but we survived and Sam was worth it.'

Sean, 26

'The first six weeks were really tough. There were times when Helen and I would have gladly traded everything we owned for a good night's sleep. I was worried about going back to work, but I coped. In fact I think at times it was easier for me than for Helen. She didn't get the same break from the constant demands of looking after the bub. I think it helped that we had been warned what to expect and we knew it went with the job.'

William, 25

'This is where I found the teamwork approach really helped. You can't predict what your baby's sleep pattern will be like – there are so many experts and books around to give you what I have come to call "gratuitous advice". Neither of us had very much unbroken extended sleep (you know, the regular seven or eight hours experts all tell us we need to be healthy) in the first two months. Harry was very erratic in his sleep patterns and he cried a lot – well it seemed like a lot to us until we traded stories with other parents. We were always getting up to him. When he was about three months, we worked out a bit of a roster system (this wasn't much good for our love life). Sharon would take the evening shift and I would take the early morning shift. So if Harry wouldn't settle after a feed from about 3 a.m. onwards, I would get up to be with him. It was my job as part of the team. This worked out very well in the long run – I still take the early mornings and really enjoy my time with him before I go to work. You might say it is my bonding time. Harry and I, milk, cereal, toast and coffee. What a mess we get into sometimes.'

Andrew, 40

'I used to love getting up in the mornings, having a shower, reading the paper over breakfast, listening to the news on the radio – getting in touch with the world and enjoying my personal space. I learnt this from my dad – he always seemed to have time to enjoy those little things in life. The only thing that was missing is the cigarette he used to have and thank God for that as I have read that passive smoking is not good for young babies. That has all changed now – life of a morning is go, go, go; Sara asleep, Sara awake, preparing for the day, sorting out Sara's clothes to take to childcare, feeding, changing nappies, dressing. I might be

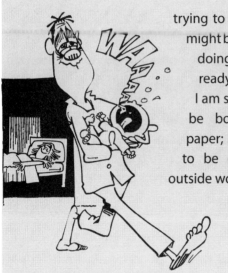

trying to settle Sara and Karen might be having a shower and doing other things to get ready for work. Sometimes I am so tired I couldn't even be bothered reading the paper; sometimes I seem to be on autopilot so the outside world is irrelevant to me – I wouldn't know what was happening elsewhere.'

David, 30

'I learnt to cat-nap. Whenever I can, I sit in the lounge or lie on the bed and catch as much sleep as possible. This was a surprise to me as I always thought I was a person who needed eight hours' sleep – go to bed at a certain time and get up at a certain time. I used to be like clockwork. I have adjusted, I have changed. I have also become skilled at spending time just relaxing and breathing, and have even tried meditation. It works for me. I always thought it was a load of crap.'

Peter, 26

In the early days of parent-hood, sleep deprivation can be severe on both mothers and fathers. In Chapter 6 there is a detailed discussion on sleep, accompanied by some survival strategies. It is important to know that parents do survive the disruption to their sleep. Probably the best thing to keep in mind is that *nothing lasts forever* – a baby who is sleeping through the night at three months might suddenly change this pattern a month later.

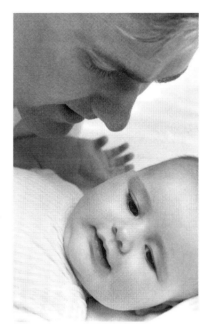

Reduced income

'At the moment we manage okay with money. I had no idea what would happen when we only had one wage. We went into a baby shop the other day and I was blown away by the cost of everything. How can things so small cost so much? We only had a small car and there was no way we were going to fit the baby and all the stuff in it, so we had to buy a bigger car. What makes it worse is that I'm only working casually. At the moment there's lots of work but if that situation changes we'll be in trouble.'

Benjamin, 28

'This hasn't been a big issue as I have a wife who is incredibly focused on money and financial planning – I am very different to this. Our mortgage payments were way, way in front, we had cash in the bank and she is generally frugal. Maybe that's a bit harsh – she is very careful with spending money. She looks for bargains (except on her own clothes: she likes nice clothes, but is not extravagant) and she uses credit cards creatively – we've never had any credit card debt. You know what I mean, she is not wasteful and is very thoughtful about what we buy for our baby.'

Luke, 31

'We make all the financial decisions together – the cot, the pram, toys and clothes. Yes, I go baby clothes shopping. I hate going shopping for clothes for my wife. Strange, isn't it? We have really struggled to make ends meet since Hetty stopped work. There were many things we would have liked to have bought for our baby, but we couldn't afford them. We have had to give up some of our luxuries and we even have a family budget now – something we had never considered before. And we both have life insurance, just in case.'

Tony, 31

'We have become bargain shoppers. We look for second-hand baby things (not mattresses) and have accepted some items from our friends. Our life was pretty basic before as we didn't have a lot of money between us, so things haven't changed much – can't think when we will be able to afford our own home. Work is a different thing. I have changed a lot there.'

Russell, 39

Finances are a worry for most first-time parents. This is especially the case if you haven't planned to have a baby. This is one thing that *has* changed over time – there are more people today who plan for a baby in their lives. In our day, there was much less planning. The financial situation just hit you. But it was also probably easier for us to survive on one income than it is for parents today. Many parents find that they need two incomes – but more commonly a full-time and a part-time income. The impact of a reduced income and tips to help you adjust are outlined in Chapter 4.

Balancing the demands of work and family life

'I didn't tell my boss about the pregnancy. I was worried how he would react. He works incredibly long hours and expects the maximum from his staff. My dad also seemed to be always working and I hardly knew him. I wanted things to be different for my child. I wanted to be there but I also wanted a career. Twelve months on, I am still struggling with these issues.'

Mario, 33

'I used to think work was the most important thing in my life. I was always there at the nursery – there was always something to do, plants to be moved, watering systems to maintain, new products to be displayed. It wasn't the money – I didn't get overtime – I just loved my job and the people I worked with. I still love my job and the people I work with, but now I am a bit more balanced in my approach. I get in early when I can, but there is more to be done at home and Jesse is so much fun now. I don't want to miss out. My boss was a bit concerned at first, but he has adjusted now too.'

Paul, 41

'You're lucky if you have a good boss. My boss didn't get it at all. She still has the same expectations as she had of me before. I took some leave early on and next thing she called me in to have a chat – a chat about my performance – she didn't think it was up to scratch. She told me I was taking too much time off and was not spending enough time in the office. I figured I was entitled to it – it is part of our company policy.'

Adam, 33

'We have a company policy for family leave, but it mainly applies to the shop floor. No-one would expect someone at my level to take leave as a father. I wouldn't feel right taking it either. As a senior manager, I have major responsibility for a major part of the business. People like me should be able to work around having a baby without it having any impact on their work performance or their attendance at work. I usually go to work at 7 a.m. and try to be home by 7 p.m. every night. My wife is there for the baby every day and I am there on the weekends. I have tried to reduce my travel as much as I can to get full weekends at home. I also try to switch off from work on the weekends. I can't do that during the week.'

Brett, 29

'You know that is a skill I have learnt, and I think I have perfected it. I am now able to switch off at home and focus on what is happening. It was hard at first, but I persisted. I found I was coming home to my Sharon and Annabelle who were both exhausted and looking forward to my walking in the door. My previous pattern of simply walking in and downloading all that had happened at work, expecting a drink and food and a receptive ear, didn't work any more. I found that I needed to provide the energy – I needed to be upbeat, to change the mood. How did I do this? I started at work. I spent the last half-hour clearing my desk and my head. I then phoned home to check on how things were and whether I needed to stop to buy anything. When I walked in the door I was ready to focus on Sharon and Annabelle.'

Frank, 26

'Sounds like you have a lot of control over your job. I work shift work, twelve hours on and twelve hours off on a rotating basis. This pattern, whether I work day or night, varies every couple of weeks. I come home totally exhausted, and this can be either at 7.30 in the morning or 7.30 in the evening. There's not much I can do about work – it is a physical thing, it is constant, and it is draining physically and emotionally. I often come home a complete wreck. What the baby has done for me, though, is she has stopped me drinking so much. Before Fiona arrived, I used to drink quite a bit on my days off. Sally had a full-time job and so I had a lot of time to myself.'

Hamish, 30

Balancing work and family life continues to be a challenge for many fathers, even though many workplaces have family friendly policies and some provide paid paternity leave. Increasingly, it is also an issue for women, because more mothers of young children are in the paid workforce today. In Chapter 9 we consider these challenges and give some ideas to help you balance the demands of work and family life.

Impact on the relationship with your partner

'I was worried that our relationship would change. We had a great life with just the two of us. Don't get me wrong, I was looking forward to being a dad and doing things as a family. It's just that I guess I thought it would be harder to find time as a couple. One of my friends told me I could forget about sex for the first few months. We both enjoy making love and I figured I would miss it if that happened – and it did! The bottom line is, the baby was the most important part of our life for quite a while.'

Michael, 42

'I forgot to mention the positive thing about shift work – our sex life has improved out of sight. On the days I have off, I am around all the time. It is amazing what you can fit in when a baby is asleep!'

Hamish, 30

'Mate, think yourself lucky. I don't know what a sex life is! I have tried everything, I have become the most romantic bloke I have ever known. But it still hasn't changed things. She has no interest in it at all, even after twelve months.'

Sam, 24

'I had somewhat the same experience – but mine only lasted for six months. It was hard, but I decided to confront the issue as I found that I was becoming more and more frustrated, angry and resentful. I had also seen my sister and her husband struggle with this issue. At times they were openly hostile to each other when we were there, and it was very uncomfortable. They never said anything, but I think they eventually went to counselling. But it was too late – they have now broken up. I decided one night after dinner, when we were both in a good mood, to talk about how we could improve our relationship and our respective needs. Yes, I actually did this. I never thought I had it in me. I remembered that I had been to a couple of communication courses at work and went and found my notes. There were things in there about using "I statements", being empathetic, not blaming, etc. I can't say

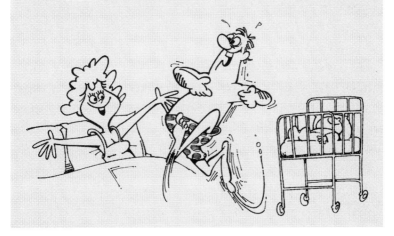

that what I did was best practice, but it did help. It opened up the discussion in a non-threatening way and as a result we both changed our behaviour towards each other.'

Anthony, 25

'I tried that, and it didn't work – maybe I wasn't as good at it as you were. What I found worked for me was to take responsibility for the relationship. I planned outings together, I organised the babysitters, I came home with flowers. It was the outings – what I began to call our personal dates, back to our courting days – that had the biggest impact.'

Nathan, 34

It is clear from both research and our experience that becoming a parent does impact on your relationship with your partner, both in terms of the quality of the relationship and the amount of time spent together. The baby can also introduce new points of tension: for example, the focus may be on what the baby needs – a feed, a longer sleep, a nappy change. We also know that how we are as a couple will affect how we parent. One of the best predictors of child wellbeing is the quality of the relationship between the mother and father. Keeping your relationship on track in your fatherhood journey is extremely important – and at times very, very difficult. Many men find that improving their communication skills helps. We provide some suggestions below on how to achieve this. We will have another look at making time for your relationship in Chapter 9.

Good communication is the key

If we had to choose the most important item in your repertoire for managing family life and fatherhood, it would be good communication. Remember when you first met your partner, and the excitement of sharing ideas, dreams and experiences? It was the communication as much as anything that brought you together as a couple. It was through communication that you got to know each other and started a relationship.

> 'We both wanted to travel. I can remember how we would lay out maps of different countries and talk for hours planning trips together. There was something magical about sharing our dreams. We never seemed to run out of things to say to each other. We would talk when we were together, then ring each other and talk some more. They were great times. The more I found out about Helen, the more I loved her.'
>
> Richard, 38

Communication was important then – and it's important now. In the following chapters we continually refer to the value of planning and the importance of good communication, but in the meantime there are some tips below that should help. The opportunity is there for you to develop a genuine team approach to parenting.

What can you do?

- Reframe the way you think about your relationship. You can't expect to change your partner's behaviour, but you *can* work to improve the quality of your relationship by changing your own behaviour.

- Develop a positive approach to your relationship, and make more positive, affirming comments (e.g. 'Thank you', 'I love the way you look at James', 'You are a great mother').
- Acknowledge your partner's issues and concerns (e.g. 'I can see that Jane not having a regular sleep pattern is bothering you').
- Be active in your listening: be attentive, maintain eye contact and ask questions to clarify (e.g. 'I hear what you are saying. Do you have any other concerns?').
- Make suggestions about what could be changed, what new strategies you could try, what you could do.
- Address any conflict in your relationship as soon as it arises – don't let it 'fester'. If you have an issue or a problem but you find it difficult to talk about, consider using the 'I statement' approach. It can really make a difference. The technique involves:
  - *Stating the problem*: '**When** you criticise me for my approach to putting James to sleep …'
  - *Expressing your feelings*: '**I feel** incompetent as a parent …'
  - *Stating why it is a problem*: '**Because** I think my contribution is not valued.'
  - *Asking for what you want*: '**What** I would like is the opportunity to put James to sleep, my way.'
- Look for opportunities to share positive experiences with your partner, like going out to dinner; this can allow you to have more open discussions about issues and concerns.

> • Set aside some time each day to sit and have a chat –
> to share the little things that each of you experienced
> during the day.

Preparing for the journey of your life

In the following chapters we provide information on what babies
need and on how to cope when baby comes home. We will also
discuss the important role you can play in the development of
your child.

The transition to parenthood is a major life change. It not
only brings the challenges outlined above but also times of
excitement, joy and discovery.

> 'I can't wait to have an excuse to regularly browse in toy-
> shops. I'm looking forward to seeing my baby grow – taking
> the first step, the first words, and of course the first smile. I
> will enjoy doing things as a family. Christmas and birthdays
> will take on new meaning – seeing the excitement when
> my child opens a present or discovers something new. I
> can't wait for the privilege of doing all I can to help my
> baby grow into a happy and much-loved child.'
>
> Mark, 28

How you adjust to being a dad will be influenced by your life
experiences, your current circumstances, and *how you prepare.*

> 'Professionally and personally, I recognised the importance
> of planning for the journey of fatherhood. Before my first

child was born I asked myself if I would be a good dad. I had my dream or vision of how I wanted things to be but questioned if I could make it happen.

Professionally, I have worked with many prospective new parents with similar dreams and doubts. I have also recognised the difference it makes if couples spend time planning together before the baby is born. It doesn't guarantee eight hours' sleep. It doesn't remove the sometimes overwhelming feeling of responsibility in caring for a baby. What it does do is increase the chance that you will face the challenges together. Working as a team makes a difference.'

Tony White

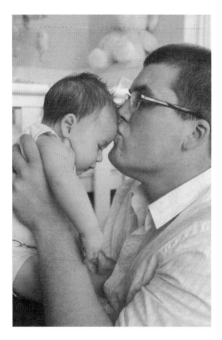

Pregnancy is an ideal time for planning. It is a time to consider how you can achieve your dreams and meet the challenges of being a dad. Planning is not a complicated process. It requires information and communication.

In the chapters ahead we will accompany you through pregnancy, birth and the early stages of parenting, and we will provide information and options to support you and your partner in planning your journey.

At all stages we will consider the questions that are frequently asked regarding the challenges that go with being a parent. Some fathers find it helpful to take the information and through communication with their partner develop a 'team plan' for each stage of their life as parents. This may work for you too.

Summary

★ Both mothers and fathers experience similar challenges in the transition to parenthood.
★ One of the major challenges is adapting to the changes in your individual lives and your life as a couple.
★ The most critical changes include increased responsibility, loss of time for leisure activities and social interactions with friends, getting used to different sleep and daily habits, managing on a reduced income, balancing life and work commitments, and dealing with the impact the arrival of a child has on your relationship.
★ Planning to spend time together as a couple and using effective communication skills are critical in ensuring the long-term wellbeing of your relationship.

4 Pregnancy

In this chapter we join you as you prepare for being a dad. Pregnancy is more than the beginning of life for your baby. It is an opportunity to share the experiences with your partner and plan for your life as parents. We will provide information on what will happen to your baby and your partner during the pregnancy and answer questions frequently asked by expectant dads. You will also hear from Carol and Paul about their experiences.

So, let's start the journey.

The beginning

You have just heard those magic words from your partner – 'I'm pregnant'.

How do you feel about the news that you are going to be a dad?

'It was really strange. My immediate reaction was to ask her if she should be standing. I took her in my arms and kept saying, "That's great, that's fantastic." I know I felt excited but I also had these strong feelings of wanting to keep her and the baby safe. It was later that other stuff started to go through my head. Will the baby be okay? How will we be able to afford a baby? What will it mean for us? Will Carol change? Will we still be able to make love? Will I be a good dad? I didn't mention any of this to Carol as I thought she may think I didn't want the baby.'

Paul, 29

Men experience a range of emotions and thoughts when faced with the reality of becoming a dad. This is not because they are men. It is because they are human and are facing a major life change.

Your partner is not immune either to the possibility of feeling anxious or apprehensive about becoming a parent.

> 'When I told Paul, I knew he was happy. I didn't tell him I was scared. I thought about a miscarriage. I wondered how I could keep the baby healthy. Would the alcohol I had last week affect the baby? How would I cope with the pain of giving birth? I also started worrying about our relationship. We had a great life together and I didn't want to lose that. Having a baby is supposed to be so natural for women.'
>
> Carol, 28

As with any major change, it can take time to find your bearings. Think about when you started a new job. At first it was probably confusing. What was expected of you? How would you know if you were going okay? It takes time to adjust. How you cope will not only depend on your commitment, but also on effective communication and appropriate information.

Let's start with what happens during pregnancy and what you need to do.

Expand your team

It's time to bring in the health professional – the first new member of your team.

As soon as the pregnancy is confirmed, you need to consider your health care options. Who will monitor the progress of the pregnancy? There is a range of health professionals – general practitioners, obstetricians, midwives – who can provide ongoing care during pregnancy.

If your partner has a local doctor she knows and trusts, it is a good idea to start there. They will be aware of her health history and the available options, which will help them provide the best advice. The person you choose will become an important member of your team until after the baby is born. Once the care decision is made, you will be booked in for an initial appointment.

What can you do?

Attending the appointment *together* is an option to consider. It is a chance to meet the new member of your team and to demonstrate your commitment to being involved from the beginning.

With your partner, make a list of questions you want answered. Write them down and take them with you. Ask some of the questions. Too often health professionals focus entirely on the mum-to-be and ignore your interest and importance in this great journey.

'I went with Carol for our first appointment with the obstetrician. He looked at me and said, "Your job is done now, Paul." I wasn't impressed. I made sure I asked some questions but he directed all his answers to Carol. It was as if I wasn't there. I kept going to appointments and I guess he got used to me. He started asking me some questions and seemed interested in what I said and how I was feeling. It felt good to be included.'

Paul, 29

If you have any questions or issues between appointments, write them down. Your selected carer will provide a list of possible complications and how you can identify them. If you or your partner have any concerns, ring up your health professional immediately.

Inform yourself

Your chosen doctor or midwife will be able to provide information on all aspects of the pregnancy. This will include what to expect, what will help, and the risk factors for your partner and baby. You will also be given a schedule for visits and any proposed screening or testing procedures.

There are numerous other sources of information about changes during pregnancy. In case your appetite for knowledge goes beyond what we provide here, we have included additional resources at the back of this book.

Let's start with a broad outline of what to expect during pregnancy.

The first trimester (conception to 14 weeks)

From the moment of conception, a single cell begins an amazing journey to become your baby. The journey is usually divided into three sections called trimesters. Each trimester lasts approximately three months.

What's happening to your baby?

In the first three months your baby has four name changes and sets up house in your partner's uterus. The *zygote* (name one) is the single cell formed from the partnership of sperm and egg. It immediately starts multiplying and begins a trip down the fallopian tube to the uterus. On its way it becomes a group of cells known as a *blastocyst* (name two). It then commences the job of setting up house. To do this it attaches to the wall of the uterus. Then things really start happening. The blastocyst develops into an *embryo* (name three) and a life support system called the *placenta*.

Your baby now goes about the job of setting up a living space. The 'room' is called the *amniotic sac* and your baby surrounds himself with fluid. The sac is set at a constant and comfortable temperature and provides plenty of room for growth and movement. As yet no television has been provided.

Once again your baby goes for a name change. At about nine weeks he decides on *foetus* (name four), which is the name he then keeps until birth. Incredibly, by this stage, most of the baby's major organs and structures have been formed.

During the first three months, the placenta develops an incredible capacity to supply oxygen and nutrients from your partner to the baby via the umbilical cord. It also transfers waste products from the baby and provides a barrier to many bacteria.

In the first trimester your baby has established the groundwork for growth.

FASCINATING FACTS ABOUT BABIES

By the end of the first trimester, your baby is about 8 centimetres long and weighs nearly 3 grams. He can do a number of things, including smile and move legs, arms, fingers and toes. His sex can be determined and he can urinate.

What's happening to your partner?

Throughout the pregnancy, your partner is undergoing changes to accommodate the growing demands of your baby and to prepare for the birth. In the first trimester an influx of new hormones causes most of the physical changes. It may be that the only perceptible body changes relate to her breasts and a small weight variation. Breasts will get bigger and they will become increasingly tender, with some possible darkening around the nipples.

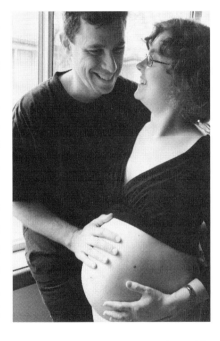

There is also a good possibility of some uncomfortable side effects. These may include nausea or 'morning sickness'; tiredness; constipation; frequent urination; aches and pains; changes to her sense of smell; and a 'metallic taste' in her mouth.

Many women also experience emotional changes in the first trimester. These may include mood swings and anxiety caused by a combination of hormonal changes and adjustment to the pregnancy.

> 'A couple of months into the pregnancy Carol was having a rough time. She seemed to be either vomiting or saying she was going to be sick. Even the smell of some food set her off. The other thing that got to me was how her moods would suddenly change for no apparent reason. We could be watching the news and she would start crying. At first, I kept asking what was wrong but she didn't know. I learned that the best thing to do was comfort her and wait for it to pass. Our sex life was pretty dramatic as well. One minute she'd say, "I want you now – immediately", and at other times I'd try to get friendly and she'd glare at me and say, "You've got to be joking". I'm telling you, this pregnancy stuff took some getting used to.'
>
> Paul, 29

What will help your partner and baby?

There is no doubt that the health and wellbeing of your partner is critical to your baby's health and development. Diet and exercise are very important, and any risk factors should be reduced. But what is often forgotten is the importance of *your* health to your baby. How you look after yourself is important at all stages of your fatherhood journey. Now is a great time to examine your lifestyle and, if necessary, make some changes in the interests of your health and your family.

'When I found out I was going to be a dad, I made some changes. I gave up smoking, booked in for a medical check-up, bought smoke detectors and took out some life insurance. I wanted my baby to be safe and secure and I wanted to be around to watch him grow.'

Paul, 29

A healthy diet

'We both worked and meals were sometimes a problem. We would often miss breakfast and have takeaway at night. Then we would get health conscious and have regular meals and watch what we ate. I guess the thing is we weren't consistent. When Carol and I found a diet recommended for pregnancy, it consisted mainly of food we ate during our "good times". We decided to give it a go, and we actually planned what to eat on a weekly basis. The thing that kept us going was the baby. We had to make some changes when Carol decided suddenly that she hated chicken. Then she hated red meat – couldn't even stand the sight of it. With all the changes I think we did pretty well. In fact I think I lost more weight than Carol put on during the pregnancy. Most importantly, the baby seems to have thrived.'

Paul, 29

What we eat affects our health. During pregnancy it is important to consider the effect of diet on both your partner and your baby. There are numerous diets recommended for pregnancy – all are based on principles that support general health, and they also recognise the nutritional needs of a mother and baby during pregnancy. The right diet can even help reduce some of the uncomfortable symptoms that pregnant women may experience. Your health professional should be able to recommend a diet that takes your partner's particular health needs into consideration.

What can you do?

A healthy diet will benefit your partner, your baby and *you*. This doesn't mean that you have to give up all your 'unhealthy' treats. What it means is that any changes you make that support your partner's efforts will help your baby.

Regular exercise

'Carol and I both went to the gym. She was really into aerobics. When we found out she was pregnant, she was worried about having to give it up.

I suggested that she talk to the people at the gym and ask if they could put her in a class that would suit. In the second half of the pregnancy she developed some problems and the doctor recommended that she stop aerobics, so we started walking. I enjoyed doing it together, and it was a great time to talk.'

Paul, 29

Exercise, like a good diet, will help your partner and the baby. The best type of exercise will depend on your partner's general health and her activity level before the pregnancy. Extreme sports are not recommended, so encourage her to give up the bungee jumping until the baby is born! Moderate exercise is good for both your partner and your baby. It will help her body deal with the demands of pregnancy and birth. Walking and swimming are excellent. If you have a different routine in mind, that's great, but run it past your health professional to be on the safe side.

One type of exercise you and your partner will hear about during the pregnancy is to do with the *pelvic floor muscles*. These muscles play an important role during the birth. They also provide support for the pelvic organs and are important in bladder and bowel control. The pelvic floor muscles and ligaments come under pressure during the birth, which can affect future bladder control. The exercises are not complicated, but they need to be done regularly to be effective.

What can you do?

Whether you are keen on exercise or not, it may be necessary to adjust your thinking so that you can provide support and encouragement to your partner. It is often easier to maintain a regular exercise program if you are doing it with someone else. It also helps if you commit to a regular time to do it together. Encourage your partner to do the recommended pelvic floor exercises; they will help with the birth and may prevent future problems of incontinence. Do them with her, as there are also benefits for your future bladder control.

Being aware of risk factors

The list of risk factors for the pregnancy will depend on your partner's health. However, some risk factors are critical to all pregnancies. These include smoking, alcohol and a large number of pharmaceutical drugs. We talked earlier in the chapter about the placenta's role of transferring nutrients from your partner to the baby. While it does this very effectively, it can also transfer many harmful substances.

Smoking can affect your baby's growth and lead to a lower birth weight. It is also associated with increased chances of respiratory problems after your baby is born. Exposure to 'passive smoke' can lead to the same outcomes.

Alcohol crosses the placenta easily, in the same concentration that exists in your partner's bloodstream. Excessive alcohol intake causes growth problems and may even lead to birth defects. The impact of alcohol on your baby is related to the amount your partner drinks, but we do not know what amount of alcohol is safe during pregnancy. For this reason, most health professionals recommend total abstinence throughout the pregnancy.

'We didn't drink a lot, but it was pretty regular. I'd have a few beers and Carol would have some wine each night when we got home from work. Sometimes on the weekend we would drink more than that, with friends. We never saw it as a problem until we found out Carol was pregnant. We talked about the information we had on the effects of alcohol on our baby. It was pretty serious. Carol stopped drinking immediately. I decided to stop drinking during the week. I still had a couple of beers at the weekend – but only a couple. When my mates questioned me about my "cutting back", I'd just say that you have to be careful when you're pregnant.'

Paul, 29

There are many other legal and illegal drugs that can affect your baby. It is strongly recommended that no drugs be taken during pregnancy – even common, over-the-counter medications for minor complaints – without checking with your health professional or pharmacist.

There are other risks involving lifestyle and exposure to certain environmental factors (such as household and gardening chemicals). Check with your health professional, but if you are still in doubt – don't.

What can you do?

Find out the risk factors for your partner and baby during pregnancy, and discuss any issues with your partner.

If she smokes, support any attempt to quit or reduce the amount. Most women stop smoking during pregnancy, but some find it very difficult. Knowing the risks is a definite incentive. Having a supportive partner also helps. Discuss it and together plan a smoke-free environment for your baby. Work with her to make the plan a reality.

Of course, if *you* smoke, one option is to stop. If you can't, at least ensure that you smoke outside the house. It's not the best answer for you but at least the baby will be spared the passive smoke.

A similar strategy could work regarding alcohol. If it is an issue, support your partner in her attempts to cut out or reduce the amount of alcohol she consumes. In terms of teamwork, it would be great if you did this together.

The second trimester (15 to 27 weeks)

This is a much safer zone for the baby. In this three-month period your baby quickly builds on the foundations of the first trimester. Having established a comfortable living space with a continuing supply of nourishment, your baby 'goes for growth'.

What's happening to your baby?

Realising that his skin is wrinkling from the long soak in liquid, your baby covers himself with a protective cream called *vernix caseosa*. To get it to stay on, your baby grows fine downy hair on his arms, legs and back. Thankfully the hair gradually disappears after birth.

The second trimester is a great time for hair growth; it also starts to appear on your baby's head, and the eyelashes and eyebrows grow too. This is the time when nails appear on fingers and toes. It is also the time when your baby starts to exercise. He stretches, rolls and even has a go at sucking his thumb. Your partner may start to feel the movement (called *quickening*) from as early as the fifth month. Many new mums initially find it hard to detect, but they definitely get the message after the baby has practised some 'rock 'n' roll'.

Your baby also develops his sense of hearing during this period; and toward the end of the second trimester he opens his eyes. Still no television!

The organs have grown and matured so much by now that intensive care babies can survive if born at the end of the second trimester.

What's happening to your partner?

For many women this is the most enjoyable time of pregnancy. With luck, the side effects experienced in the first trimester reduce. The mood swings are fewer, nausea decreases or disappears, and your partner will probably feel physically well – most of the time. We have to warn you that there is no guarantee. Every pregnancy is different.

The physical changes become more obvious. The uterus starts to move above the pelvic area and settles near your partner's navel. Her belly will expand to accommodate the growing uterus. For most women the second trimester means they start to 'look' pregnant.

The nutritional demands of the baby lead to an increase in your partner's blood flow. This is good for the baby, but the results for your partner are mixed. She could find that her hair and nails grow more quickly, and that she has more sensitive gums.

This is the time when people start to describe your partner as 'radiant'. For some reason everyone also thinks they have the right to touch her belly. Stay calm. It probably comes from some ancient ritual carried out because people felt positive and excited about the new life. It can, however, be a nuisance to your partner.

What will help your partner and baby?

In the first trimester you achieved a lot. Working with your partner as you adjusted to pregnancy has set you up for the challenges ahead. You have discussed diet, exercise and risk factors. You have hopefully been able to attend some appointments with your health professional along with your partner. This has been a challenging time for both of you. It is important to acknowledge what you have achieved.

Now, what can you achieve in the second trimester?

Building a connection with your baby

Remember the early days with your partner, and the mystery and excitement of a new relationship? Well, this is another new relationship.

In the first trimester you found out about your baby. You then worked with your partner to ensure the safest possible transition to the more secure world of the second trimester. Now you have the chance to build on this by making direct contact with your baby.

Until now your baby has been a series of symptoms. The only way you knew that he existed was through what you were told, what you read or what you imagined. This changes in the second trimester, as it is usual (though not compulsory) for the woman to have an ultrasound scan during this period. This will be your *first direct contact* – seeing the baby-to-be.

> 'I couldn't believe it. There was my baby on a television screen. It all seemed so unreal up to that point. Now my baby was real. It was like I was a parent already. It wasn't pretty but it was bloody beautiful. They said they could probably tell us if it was a boy or a girl. We didn't want to know. We just wanted to be sure it was all there. I mean that it was okay.'
>
> Paul, 29

The *second direct contact* will be when the baby moves.

> 'Carol said she could feel the baby moving. I put my hand on her bump but couldn't feel anything. This happened for two days. Then I felt it. I loved it when the baby was moving. We would just sit there together and be amazed. I could put my head on her stomach and feel the kicks and hear the heartbeat.'
>
> Paul, 29

The *third direct contact* will be when the baby can hear.

'They say that if you talk to your baby, it can hear you. Not only that, but they reckon your baby gets used to your voice and can recognise it when they are born. I not only talked, I read stories to her and kept her up to date with the football scores! There were times when I'm sure that she stopped moving when I started talking.'

Paul, 29

This is a magic way to develop a new relationship.

Working as a team with your partner

To work well as a team, you need to plan and you also need to communicate. In the first trimester you probably discussed a number of issues with your partner. You

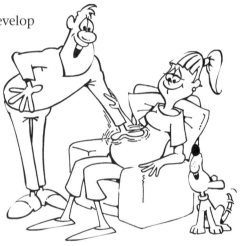

were interested enough to find out what was happening to her. You showed interest and concern for the baby. The message to your partner was: *'this is our baby'*. Sharing the responsibility for your baby is a great basis for a lifelong partnership in the journey ahead. It will both benefit your baby *and* strengthen your relationship with your partner.

So continue with the communication. There are still many things to discuss and plan, including issues relating to finance, antenatal education classes, and your relationship. Let's start by discussing finances.

Planning your finances

'We planned to have the baby but we didn't really talk much about the money side of things. Now that Carol is pregnant, I'm starting to worry. It really hit home when Carol took me into a baby shop. I was shocked at what babies need and how much it cost. With just the two of us we coped with all our expenses and were able to put a bit aside. But that was on two wages. Carol wants to be at home for at least the first twelve months. I want that too but I don't know if we can afford it.'

Paul, 29

The first thing to do is your homework:

★ Check out any benefits or entitlements provided for parents.

★ Find out what is available from your employers. Leave provisions vary from area to area and often from job to job. Check with your boss or the human resources section of your organisation. If possible, get your entitlements in writing.

★ Check out whether you are eligible for benefits from the government – again, get it in writing. At the same time, you may like to collect the application forms you will need.

Now that you have the information at hand, you can discuss and plan.

A basic but effective approach to financial planning is to lay out both your projected income and your future costs. If this appears daunting, seek assistance from someone with the necessary expertise. Banks are often very willing to help and usually don't charge for this service. The time you devote to financial planning during the pregnancy will help to prevent anxiety after the baby is born.

You also need to take into account what you will need for your baby. The range of clothes and equipment on the market is endless. Before you choose anything, talk to friends and family members about their experiences. What did they find was essential?

Make a list of essentials and shop around. If your budget is tight, consider alternatives. Try second-hand stores or garage sales, and ask friends and family members. It is amazing how many people keep prams, cots and other goodies in their attic or garage. They are usually only too happy to let you use them. If new is your preference, then still shop around. Prices do vary enormously.

Whether the baby equipment is new or used, safety is a major consideration. Check that it complies with the relevant standards. (We cover this in more detail in Chapter 7.)

Hidden financial issue

'It felt strange after I left work. I wasn't earning my own money. I was so used to having my money. Even though we pooled our income and had a joint bank account, it was like I had lost some independence.'

Carol, 28

It is common for women to feel a loss of independence when they leave work. Fathers who assume the primary care role for their children often report the same experience. Like many other areas in a relationship, it is often enough to acknowledge the feelings. In a team approach, it is helpful to discuss the issue without thinking you have to find a magic solution.

Attending antenatal classes

Your health professional will tell you about the antenatal education classes held in your area. They are usually offered by hospitals, local health centres or private midwives.

This is a chance to obtain information, ask questions and, importantly, to share experiences with other prospective parents. The reality is that the content and style of the classes are determined by the skills, training and attitudes of the educator.

At antenatal classes you should expect to be acknowledged as important. This means you should be included in all aspects of the program. Your input should be valued and encouraged. Too often fathers-to-be are referred to and treated as a 'support person'.

> 'She kept calling me a support person. I wanted to stand up and say – "I'm the dad". "Support person" made me feel second rate, unimportant – like I was just some sort of back-up. I'm not.'
>
> Paul, 29

Here you are starting to think, feel and act like a father and someone is changing your role back to that of 'extra'. Imagine if your partner was referred to as an 'incubator'! You would both be offended – and rightly so. It is important that the language used is respectful and inclusive of all members of the class.

You may choose to challenge or ignore the 'support person' description. Whatever you decide, act as a partner, a father-to-be and a key member of the team.

Classes should include sessions on parenting. The better classes will not just focus on 'birth plans', pain control and breathing exercises. They will include discussion with couples about their fears, vision and expectations of the birth and their role as parents.

Feedback shows that prospective parents are eager to know what will happen when the baby comes home and how it will affect their relationship. They are also interested in what support is available after the birth.

Antenatal classes are also an excellent opportunity to discuss issues we have previously raised, including the expectations placed on both mothers and fathers.

It is a mistake to believe that the focus at antenatal classes should be entirely on the birth.

There is increasing evidence that classes directed at improving relationships during pregnancy have a positive effect – not only on the couple relationship but on the father's involvement with their child.

'It was good getting information about the pregnancy and the birth but they told us very little about how to look after the baby when we took it home.

Carol and I both wanted some practical stuff on what to expect and how to deal with it. We knew our lives were going to change big time. It would have been great to have had a chance to discuss this with the other people in the group.'

Paul, 29

It is also necessary that educators recognise and value the importance of the social support developed in these classes. When we talked about team parenting earlier, we mentioned that the team should include others, not just you and your partner. Your team may include family members and friends, but it could also include the people you meet in the antenatal classes. They can provide valuable support simply because they are experiencing the same changes as you. They will understand.

These classes provide an opportunity for prospective parents to share the experiences, dreams and fears of this great journey in safety. For some parents-to-be this is the first time since school that they have been in a group situation. At first it can be daunting.

If the educator has good facilitation skills, it will become easier as the classes progress. In fact, feedback from classes shows that sharing is at least as important as the information you receive. The result could be increased support of your role as parents.

> 'I didn't know what to expect when I first entered that room full of strangers. The educator made us feel welcome and by the third week I was looking forward to going. We had a topic to discuss each week. After a few weeks I realised that the mums didn't know everything. I started to feel comfortable – not stupid – and got a lot out of talking with other group members. We even gave our group a name – "Sleepers" – as there wasn't one morning person in our group. The thing I enjoyed most about the classes was being with the other members of our group, people I'd never met before, but we had one very important thing in common – having a baby.'
>
> Paul, 29

Our experience tells us that the bond of sharing this life change is powerful. It can cut across differences in life experiences and current circumstances.

It is a good idea to share phone numbers and organise a 'reunion' some time after the babies are born. It is amazing how often groups formed in antenatal classes continue to meet well after the birth of their first baby.

'We got together for a "reunion" about six weeks after the last baby was born. It was great catching up with the other people from the class. The stories varied, but we had a lot in common. I enjoyed the chance to talk "babies" with other dads. I realised that the way we were struggling was normal – it made me feel we weren't alone. Since the reunion we have kept in contact with most of the people from the class. Some we see regularly. Some we only see at a six-monthly gathering in a local park. We have been doing this for about five years. When our first-born was about two I used to meet some of the dads at a playground on Saturday morning. We'd then go and have coffee. I looked forward to it.'

Paul, 29

FASCINATING FACTS ABOUT BABIES

By the end of the second trimester your baby is up to 36 centimetres long and weighs up to 900 grams. His eyes are open and he can hear. He has hair, eyelashes and eyebrows and is able to roll over.

The third trimester (28 to 40 weeks)

Your baby is really getting his act together for the big day. This is the time when the brain grows rapidly, senses are fine-tuned and sight improves so that your baby can see a bright light 'through' your partner's stomach.

What's happening to your baby?

★ In the last month before birth, your baby's hearing is as good as that of a newborn. He will get used to regular noises and may recognise those same sounds after birth. Because it would be familiar, your favourite music could prove to be a useful pacifier when needed. The same applies to your voice.

★ In the first half of the third trimester, baby is really giving your partner's stomach a workout. Lightly patting the 'bump' can sometimes get a response.

★ As the baby continues to grow, space in the uterus is at a premium. This could lead to his movements changing and becoming less 'violent' towards the end of the pregnancy.

★ The baby now has more obvious times of sleep and activity. This may or may not fit in with your partner's routine.

★ In preparing for life in the 'big bad world', your baby practises breathing exercises – not actual breathing, but the chest and diaphragm start getting ready for the first breath.

★ Also in preparation for the big day, your baby takes in some antibodies through the placenta. This provides short-term protection from diseases to which your partner is immune.

★ In this trimester your baby moves into position for birth. For most, this is head down. Some stubbornly sit on their bum, which is known as the breech position.

★ Your baby will put on some 'fat' and his skin will become less wrinkly – or maybe baby just grows into his skin.

What's happening to your partner?

As the baby continues growing, the uterus moves up toward the breasts. This can place pressure on your partner's ribs and diaphragm, and may cause discomfort and shortness of breath. As the baby moves into its preferred position for birth, the pressure in the rib area should decrease.

There are still a number of side effects that may occur as your partner's body and the baby prepare for the big day. These could include varicose veins, backache, haemorrhoids, swollen ankles, increased urination and heartburn. Your partner may also develop 'stretch marks' on her stomach, thighs or breasts.

As the baby's weight increases, this will present challenges in standing, moving and finding a comfortable position – day and night.

The approach of the due date can lead to increased concern regarding the health of the baby and the actual birth process – a mixture of wanting it to be over and apprehension about how your partner and the baby will cope. This is also the time when she is most likely to get a seat on the bus!

In the third trimester, it is common to become increasingly protective towards your partner and the baby.

'The last six weeks were not easy for Carol. She wasn't sleeping well and her back was giving her hell. I started to really worry that something would go wrong. She didn't complain but would often go quiet. I tried to help by massaging her back and legs. I bought a special pillow to help her get comfortable. I helped as much as I could. The hard part was that there wasn't anything I could do to make the time go quicker.'

Paul, 29

What will help your partner and baby?

There is no doubt that your practical help and support are important. It is also true that most men feel they want to do more to take away the discomfort of the last part of pregnancy.

Well, here's something *more* you can do.

Remember that your partner is important to you as a person. If there was ever a time to be romantic, this is it. She is feeling uncomfortable and could have issues about her body image. Imagine how you would feel with a beach ball full of sand stuck in your stomach! It's not enough to tell her you love her – show her.

How can you show her you love her? This is a question you need to ask at all stages of your relationship, but this is one time when it is critical. Helping ease the discomfort is a great start. Being an active participant in household chores is even better. This will become critical after you have your baby!

Now let's move into second gear and bring back the romance of those early days.

Buy flowers

Taking home flowers will give the message that she is still your number one person in the world. Buying flowers is a clear message that you care about her. To really get your message across, add a card. Select something that represents love and friendship and write a simple message that conveys your feelings and makes her feel special.

Arrange special or surprise outings

Is there somewhere or something that is special for both of you? It could be anything you both associate with a good time in your relationship – a particular restaurant; a special place for a picnic; where you met.

Organise it and surprise her. The message will be clear – she is special.

Communicate with your partner

A critical part of communication is listening. Most of us probably think we are good listeners, but in reality we can be easily sucked into a common communication problem with our partners – too often we concentrate on the 'facts' in the message and ignore the 'feelings'.

Consider this. Your partner asks you, 'How will I cope with the pain?' Even basic listening skills would tell you that your partner is worried about the birth.

Here are some possible responses:

★ You reassure her. You tell her that the doctor says everything is okay and that you will be there to support her.

★ You pull out all the information on pain relief. You assure her that you will insist on a plentiful supply of pethidine and, if necessary, threaten the staff until they reduce the pain.

★ You recommend a caesarean.

All of these responses focus on the 'facts'. However, the reassurance and information may send a message like: 'You're silly to be worried.' You went for a solution. You ignored your partner's feelings.

What can you do?

This is a great opportunity to practise 'feelings before facts' – a method of communicating that is important for close relationships and teamwork. Instead of the above, try this:

'You feel scared about the pain?'

This response acknowledges how your partner is feeling. It also encourages her to expand on how she feels.

She may continue:

'I've been told some horror stories about labour. Sally told me she was in labour for twenty hours. She said she completely lost control and screamed for hours. Nothing seemed to help. I don't want to lose it. I'm not good at putting up with even a headache. I just don't know how bad it's going to be. And what if something goes wrong for the baby?'

Your partner is expressing the normal fears of a first-time mum. Fear of the unknown. Fear of dealing with certain pain. Fear of losing control. Fear that there will be something wrong with the baby.

Resist the temptation to find a solution. Start with something like 'It must be really scary for you' and follow this with a comforting cuddle.

She may continue talking. She may cry. Importantly, the sky hasn't fallen in because you didn't offer a solution. Simply expressing her fears is healthy for her.

What about how you feel?

The benefits of expressing feelings about the impending birth also apply to you.

New dads-to-be can have a number of concerns. Commonly they include:

★ Will the baby be healthy?

★ How will I cope with seeing my partner in pain?

★ How will I react during the birth?

It is interesting to note the similarities; prospective mums and dads are both worried about the unknown and about losing control.

Your feelings are equally important. Talking about them will help. Try it out on your partner. Again, it's good practice for the journey ahead.

Sex during pregnancy

Intimacy is an important part of relationships, and this does not change during pregnancy. Unless there are medical reasons preventing it, sexual intercourse may continue throughout the pregnancy. Many couples notice the impact of physical and emotional changes on how they experience intimacy. Nausea and hormonal changes in the early stages can lead to decreased desire in your partner. Her libido may rapidly increase at other stages and then be countered by physical discomfort as the birth nears. Desire in both partners can also be affected by concern for the baby. It is a time when you can explore new dimensions in sex and intimacy.

Think about the following:

- Create alternatives to maintain intimacy at those times when your partner's desire is affected by nausea and hormonal changes. Try a gentle shoulder massage and words of love, and be patient.
- Discuss different positions and activities with your partner to meet both of your sexual needs.
- Develop and practise a belief that sexual activity is part of a 24-hour approach to intimacy. Bring back some of the romance you used at the beginning of your relationship – a great investment for a long-term relationship.

- Remember that pregnancy only lasts for nine months – your relationship with your partner is for life.
- Keep a sense of humour.

This has been a time of discovery and planning. Your involvement in the pregnancy has laid the foundation for the next part of the journey – becoming a dad.

Summary

★ When you first find out that your partner is pregnant, seek out information and expand your support team.
★ There will be many changes in both your partner and your baby during each trimester of the pregnancy.
★ Useful ways of supporting your partner and baby include ensuring the health and physical wellbeing of your partner so that your baby will be healthy too; establishing a connection with your baby; planning your finances; and maintaining good communication with your partner, particularly towards the end of the pregnancy when she will really need your support.
★ Remember to care for yourself by talking to your partner about any concerns you may have.

5 Labour and birth

Following nine months of preparation, you are ready for the next stage of your journey – the birth of your baby. In this chapter we will:

* tell the stories of fathers as they recall their experiences of labour and the birth

* provide information on what's happening at each stage

* give you some ideas about how to get involved

* celebrate the arrival of your baby with you.

The presence of fathers at the birth of their children is now routine and even expected. It wasn't always this way. Until the middle of the '70s you would have been stuck in a 'waiting room', awaiting the announcement, 'Your child has been born'. Fathers were regarded as unnecessary and even a hindrance to the birthing process.

Tony: I have been involved in a number of attempts over the years to raise awareness of how important it is to include dads in the birth of their baby. Many hospitals and health professionals have accepted the benefits of including them in the process, but some have not. I still hear stories from dads who felt like intruders in the maternity or birthing units. If dads are included and encouraged to participate, it can make a difference to the birth experience of their partner and to the outcomes for their children.

The vast majority of dads are present at the birth of their first child. Some are keen. Some are apprehensive. Some are ambivalent.

'It was never in doubt. From the moment we found out Carol was pregnant, I wanted to be involved. I went to classes and read books and we made a birth plan. Carol wanted a natural birth so we practised breathing, relaxation and massage to help her in labour. She was keen not to take medication to deal with the pain.

Even though I felt prepared, I got worried when the labour started – or when I thought it had begun. Carol had a backache and started to have some contractions. At first they were irregular and seemed to ease when she moved. I'd read about the stages of labour but I still panicked. I wanted her to ring the hospital and check. She was calmer than me and wanted to wait. I made myself busy by drawing up a chart to record the contractions and we practised our breathing. About five hours later the contractions became stronger and more frequent. Then her waters broke. She rang the hospital and explained what was happening and they told us to come in.

It was a long day. Everything went as expected but it was slow. We spent a lot of time moving around and we made good use of the shower. The nurses would check on Carol but pretty well let us do our own thing. I did what I always do when I meet people I don't know. I introduced myself and asked their names. I think that made a difference in how I was treated. I had to do it again when the new shift came on – yeah, it was a long day.

Things got hectic towards the birth. The breathing didn't seem to be working and Carol didn't want to be massaged. She just wanted to hold my hand. This threw me. I wanted to do something to help. To stop the pain. I hated feeling useless.

When our little girl was born, it was the greatest moment of my life. They let me cut the cord and hold her after they had checked her out. I wouldn't have missed it for the world.'

Paul, 29

'For me it was different. I wasn't sure about being at the birth. I really didn't know how I'd react. I never said anything as I knew Sue expected me to be there and I just accepted it – but I was nervous. I mean I wanted to be there for her but I don't like hospitals. I went to a few classes and the birth film they showed scared the daylights out of me.

I guess I left most of the breathing and stuff to her and I didn't really know what to expect when she went into labour. Like Paul, I panicked when the contractions started. It was the middle of the night and I talked Sue into ringing the hospital. They talked to her for a while and suggested we ring back in a few hours. Well, in an hour I got her to ring again. I think I made her as nervous as I was. They suggested we come in but after examining her for a while they sent us home again. They told us what to look for and asked me to keep a record of the contractions. I think they just wanted to give me something to do.

It wasn't until about ten the next morning that the timing seemed to be right. We went to the hospital and this time we stayed. It still took about six hours and I tried to help Sue by doing everything the nurses suggested. Half the time I didn't understand what they were talking about. One nurse said to me, "Your baby is OP ['occipital posterior']". I thought that was a type of rum! Near the end our doctor said he was going to use the "ventouse". He pulled out this suction thing that you use to unblock drains. He then put it on the baby's head and pulled. I don't think Sue would have cared if they had brought in a tow truck. She just wanted it over. But it freaked me out. I remember at one stage Sue asked for pethidine. They said it was too late. That made me angry. If I could have found it, I would have given it to her myself and I told them so. I think they regarded me as a bloody nuisance but I just wanted them to do anything to stop the pain. I mean, that was their job.

Finally our son arrived. The cord was around his neck and they took him out of the room quickly. They didn't say anything to us and we didn't know what had happened. That was scary. They brought him back and said he was okay and I've never felt so relieved in my life. He was okay and Sue was fine – except for a few stitches.

I know they deliver thousands of babies and the mum and bub are their priorities but they should explain what's happening – in words we understand. It's a different world in there and I felt like an intruder.'

Steve, 31

'We had a planned caesarean because the baby was in the breech position – or upside down. The doctor said he could try turning the baby around by manipulating through her stomach. Helen opted for a caesar.

In a way I was glad that she didn't have to go through the pain of childbirth. I was also worried about them cutting her open.

They took her into theatre and I put on all the surgical gear – gown, mask and shoes. They gave her an epidural and I was allowed in when she was ready for the caesar.

I was told to stay up near her head and they had a sheet up so we couldn't see what was happening. By this time Helen was scared. She held my hand so tight I got a cramp. It didn't take long for our son to arrive – but it seemed like hours to me and even longer for Helen. At one stage near the end I was tempted to have a look at what was going on. They told me to stay up the other end and not look.

They took Helen into the recovery area and while she was there they checked my son and handed him to me. I've never held anything so wonderful in my life. I just stood there with a stupid grin on my face for nearly an hour. Then I took him to Helen but she was still very shaky from the operation and just wanted to know that he was okay. I guess one thing I wasn't prepared for was how long it took Helen to recover. She was in hospital for five days and still very sore when she got home. Luckily I had two weeks off work. I don't think she could have coped on her own.'

Tom, 30

'We also had a caesarean but it wasn't planned. Like Paul, I was keen to be present at the birth. I got nervous as the labour started but we did some of the things we had learned in classes. I timed the contractions and we practised relaxation. We guessed it was going to be a while before we went to the hospital so we watched one of Julie's favourite movies – *Sleepless in Seattle*. I wanted to watch *Shrek*.

The contractions became more painful and more frequent. The pain no longer eased when she moved around. We phoned the hospital and they called us in.

When we got there, everything seemed to be going well for the first few hours. We used the shower and the birth ball. I massaged Julie's feet and back as much as she wanted. Then it all changed. The contractions stopped getting stronger and weren't as regular. They started monitoring the baby regularly. After another four hours they told us the labour wasn't progressing as it should and the baby was showing signs of distress. They recommended a caesarean.

They took Julie to theatre and put me in a room the size of a large closet and told me to put on the surgical gear. They said they'd come back for me when Julie had been prepared for surgery. I guess I was in that room for about 30 minutes and it was horrible. I was worried about Julie and the baby. We had heard about caesars in the classes, but I didn't pay too much attention as we were planning a natural birth and everything was going fine in the pregnancy. Finally they came and got me.

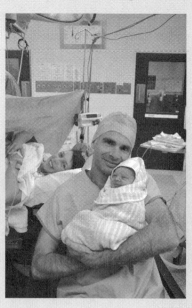

As Tom said, they told me to stay up near Julie's head and I didn't see anything. I think I squeezed her hand harder than she held mine. I seemed to go into a daze during the operation and didn't hear the first time the doctor told me what we had. Then he repeated it – "a beautiful little girl". I also got to hold her before Julie. It was wonderful.

Julie was okay but very sore for quite a while. While she was in hospital she talked to me about her disappointment. She said she felt robbed of the chance to give birth naturally. It was as if she felt it was her fault. She got upset and all I could say was I was glad that she and the baby were both well. She was worried that if we had another baby she would need another caesarean. We talked to the doctor, who told us the chances are increased but it was still possible to have a vaginal birth with the next child.'

Sam, 26

The experiences of our new dads were all very different. If you asked a hundred new parents you would probably get a hundred different stories. Labour and birth are unique experiences, and unless you have a planned caesarean, there is no way of knowing how long it will take and how you and your partner will cope. However, it helps if you have information about what is happening in labour and what you can expect at the birth.

Let's start at the beginning.

First stage of labour

How will you know your partner is in labour? In an ideal world it would go something like this:

Doctor/Midwife: 'You will start your labour on 8 June at 8.15 a.m.'

It would be a great help if your doctor or midwife could tell you exactly when labour will start. They can't. They don't even know with any certainty why it begins.

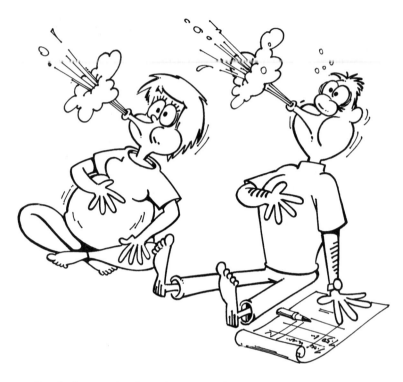

But before we look at the signs of labour, let's examine what is happening to your partner.

Your partner may experience a number of symptoms that tell you she is about to start labour. This is sometimes called pre-labour. The experience is different for each woman but commonly involves mild, irregular contractions, which usually go away if she moves.

Labour is described as starting when the contractions become regular and the intensity increases – and the pain doesn't go away when she changes position.

A *contraction* is the tightening of the muscles of the uterus. The purpose is to push the baby towards the cervix (and ultimately into the outside world). At the same time, the uterus thins out at the bottom, preparing the way for the baby. The *cervix* or neck of the uterus dilates (opens) to about 10 centimetres during labour. The uterus and the vagina then become the *birth canal*.

The first stage of labour usually takes between eight and fourteen hours for a first-time mother.

What can you do?

The best advice for pre-labour and early in the first stage is to keep both you and your partner occupied. It is suggested that you stay at or close to home and spend the time relaxing, practising breathing during the contractions, and maybe watching a movie or two. It is also a good idea to draw up a chart to record the contractions – something simple that shows how long each contraction lasts and how far apart they are, measured from the start of one to the beginning of the next. Also record any other symptoms or concerns you may have. This will not only let you know how things are going, it will be useful when you talk to your doctor or the staff at the hospital.

When should you call the doctor or hospital?

It is a good idea to ask your doctor or midwife, during the pregnancy, about *who* you should call when labour arrives. They will also give you advice about *when* to call. This is important, as they know the details of your pregnancy and there may be a reason to call if a particular symptom occurs.

As our new dads have said, the start of labour can cause anxiety in both you and your partner. Even very well-prepared couples sometimes react to the anxiety rather than to the signs. This is crunch time and most people become anxious. You are in a situation that you have never previously experienced, and the decisions you make could impact on the wellbeing of your baby. If you are going to err in your judgement, you want it to be on the side of caution.

It is most commonly recommended that you ring when contractions are becoming regular and intense. This usually means that the contractions last nearly a minute and are approximately five minutes apart. There will be no relief when your partner changes position and she will probably have difficulty talking for the duration of each contraction. But these are guidelines only, and your experience may differ.

You should also ring the doctor or hospital if your partner's membranes rupture (if her 'waters break'). Membranes surround the amniotic sac that has contained your baby during the pregnancy. When they rupture, amniotic fluid leaks from the vagina. For some women the leak may be confused with poor bladder control; for others it is a more dramatic 'gush'. Thus it may be obvious to some women and not to others. It may be a sign that labour is about to start, or it may occur during labour. It can also be accompanied by a 'bloody show' – a small amount of blood as the mucus plug that has been protecting the baby comes away. Regardless, you should ring.

Listening to the stories of new dads, and based on our experience – ring when you feel you need to.

If you are unsure about where things are up to – *ring*.

If you have questions about what is happening – *ring*.

If either you or your partner are becoming anxious – *ring*.

It is probably best if your partner makes the call. The health professional on the other end of the phone will not only want the information you have recorded but will listen carefully to your partner and make an assessment of her level of anxiety; they may even want to talk to her during a contraction to gauge the intensity. Babies being born on the way to hospital still make the papers: it is not a common event.

What should you take to the hospital?

Your partner will undoubtedly have a bag packed ready to go. It will include recommended items for the labour and her stay in hospital.

Your needs are not as great but we do suggest the following:

* Your swimsuit so that you can comfortably spend time in the shower with your partner.

* Snacks and drinks for what could be a long labour. You may be offered a drink, but don't count on the hospital supplying you with food.

* A mobile phone and money for a payphone. Hospitals have policies on the use of mobile phones in certain areas.

* A list of phone numbers of people to call after the birth. A variation on this is to ring one person who has been assigned the task of contacting the rest of those on your list. Most dads want to share the excitement personally, but having a contact person does free you up to be with your partner.

* A change of clothes is also not a bad idea. It could be a long day – or night.

There are a number of other things you may wish to take, including a camera and a portable CD player or radio. If you plan on taking anything electrical, check the hospital policy first.

Of course, take your partner!

What happens at the hospital?

Our new dads gave clear messages that what happens from the moment you arrive at the hospital will vary. Both the length and nature of the labour, what procedures are necessary and what is available will affect your experience. Your main concerns will be the wellbeing of your partner and your baby.

Think of yourself as part of the team that will care for your partner during labour and the birth. The health professionals are the experts and it is important that you accept that. You can help with the non-medical pain relief, provide encouragement and act as an interpreter or messenger between your partner and the health professionals.

In his story, Paul described how he established contact with the health professionals. His approach improves the chance that you will be included as part of the team – not treated as an extra or even a nuisance.

Introduce yourself to all the staff and find out their names. If possible, remember and use them. Like Paul, you may have to repeat this if your stay covers more than one shift.

Now that you're a member of the team, what is your role?

What you do will depend on how you prepared and, as we have said, what happens during the labour and birth process. A primary focus for you and your partner will be the issue of pain associated with labour and birth. It can't be ignored, but it can be managed.

What does non-medical pain relief involve?

All hospitals provide a range of medical and non-medical approaches to pain management. It is recommended that you visit the proposed birthing destination with your partner to find out what is available.

Most antenatal classes include a visit to the hospital. If you didn't attend classes, you can arrange a tour directly with the hospital. By doing this, you will not only discover what pain management options are available, you will familiarise yourselves with the environment. Knowing what to expect can help reduce anxiety.

If you attended antenatal classes, you will be aware of some techniques to help your partner cope with the pain of contractions. These may include breathing patterns, relaxation and massage. What helps will not only depend on the practice you put in during the pregnancy, but also on your partner and how she is coping with labour.

Massage may be acceptable and comforting to your partner in the early stages of labour. However, when the birth draws nearer, she may not want to be touched – let alone massaged. Some dads find this frustrating because, when giving a massage, at least they are doing something.

It may be that the breathing exercises you have practised provide some comfort for a while, but then your partner may lose interest. It is thought that even if breathing methods don't reduce pain, they may have some value as a distraction technique – that is, concentrating on breathing may distract your partner from the pain. This benefit is usually only experienced in the early stages. In the later stages, your partner may just want to hold your hand.

What can you do?

- Joining your partner in a shower, bath or spa will help keep her safe and make her feel more secure. Water is a very effective aid during labour. Aren't you glad you packed your swimmers?

- Unless there is a medical reason prohibiting it, your partner will be encouraged to move around during labour. It may take a while to help her find a comfortable position, and her preference may change regularly. Some positions your partner may like to try are standing, walking, rocking, sitting, and leaning on furniture. Some hospitals provide a gym ball. This allows a range of positions and can be very effective in pain management.
- Hot and cold packs can be applied to the back or abdomen. The hospital can advise you about what they have or what you can bring from home. (Ensure that hot packs are not *too* hot, as during labour they can easily burn your partner's skin without her noticing.)

The effectiveness of any form of non-medical pain relief is an individual experience. Until the time comes, you can't be sure what will work for your partner. The more options you have, the greater the chance of some relief during labour and the birth.

What about medical pain relief options?

The main options for medical pain relief are *nitrous oxide*, *pethidine* and an *epidural*.

Nitrous oxide

Also known as *laughing gas*, it is delivered through a face mask. Your partner places the mask on her face when she feels a contraction start. It is quick-acting but unfortunately does not work for all women. There is also the possibility of your partner feeling sick or even vomiting. Many a dad has reported wanting to try the mask themselves during the labour.

Pethidine

This is basically a member of the morphine group and acts as a muscle relaxant. For many women it can provide effective pain relief. It is injected and the effect lasts up to three hours. Sometimes pethidine has an impact on the baby, leading to time in the special care nursery. The timing of the pethidine in relation to the birth is a critical factor.

Epidural

With an epidural, painkilling drugs are injected into your partner's spine in the lower back area; they act to 'block' the pain of contractions. This is effective for most women but an anaesthetist is required to carry out the procedure. It takes time to work, so it is not usually recommended in the final phase leading up to the birth. For some women, there are side effects – from headache to more severe symptoms including ongoing lack of feeling in parts of their legs, which can continue for months. Your partner will probably be confined to bed once the epidural has been administered.

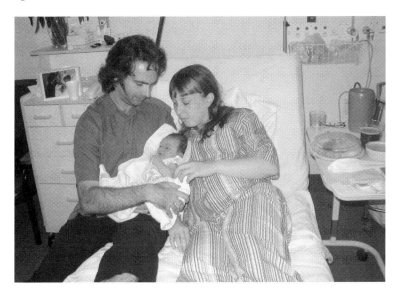

Even if you are both committed to a natural birth without medical pain relief, it is useful to know what options are available and how they work. Pain, as we have said, is a personal experience, and the most committed woman may change her mind during labour. This is her right and her choice – it is her pain.

Second stage of labour

The second stage starts when your partner's cervix is fully dilated (open). Now the role of contractions is to push the baby through the birth canal. For first-time mums this can take up to two hours, or even a little more.

As each contraction occurs, so does the urge to 'push'. The pushing moves the baby towards the exit. This is when the experts really earn their money. The midwife or doctor will coach your partner – telling her when to push and when to rest. They will also continually assess her progress.

How will you be feeling?

If ever there is a time in your life when you feel useless, this is generally it.

Many dads describe their feelings in the last stages of labour as a mixture of helplessness and anger. They feel helpless because they can't do the one thing they want to do most – stop the pain. Feelings of anger may be directed at the staff, because they also don't seem to be able to stop the pain.

> 'Up until now I really hadn't thought about how I felt just before the birth. I know I felt angry. At the time I thought it was because the doctor and nurse didn't seem to care about Sue's pain. They kept giving her instructions and

didn't respond to her distress. At one stage she screamed "Please stop it!" and they just calmly gave more instructions. I remember saying loudly, "Can't you do something?" – and they ignored me.

Talking in this group, I realise that the person I was angry with was me. I should have been able to do more for Sue. I've always felt protective towards her and would do anything to keep her safe. This time I couldn't do a damn thing. I wanted to stop the pain but I couldn't. It was rotten feeling so bloody useless.'

Steve, 31

Fathers don't often have a chance to talk about their reactions during the labour. It is rare for them to be debriefed following the birth. The focus is on the baby and the mum. Dads are often so relieved it is all over that they push their experiences to the back of their mind.

Being placed in a stressful position with no answer or no way out often produces feelings of helplessness. No-one likes feeling helpless, so the feeling can turn to anger.

What Steve has described is both common and normal. It would help if dads did have a chance to debrief – even if it were just a chance to understand what happened to them.

What can you do?

There are some things you can do:

1 **Provide encouragement.** This may not seem like much, but it can make a difference, even though your words may seem to disappear amidst all the action. Yours is a familiar voice and saying something like

'You are doing well' after each pushing session is not a waste of time.

2 **Act as an interpreter.** Translating or restating the instructions from staff can help. If you don't understand, ask for an explanation and pass on the information to your partner. Having information about what is happening and where it's all at could help both you and your partner.

3 **Stay as calm as possible.** It is not easy seeing your partner in pain. We have described some possible feelings you may experience. It will help if you can keep the feelings under control and appear calm – even if you are not. This is not easy but it may help your partner to feel that everything is okay.

Your partner may want to hold onto you – or she may not want to be touched. Be prepared for a range of reactions and go with her wishes.

What if things don't go as planned?

With variations, most births go pretty much as planned. There are, however, times when the unexpected happens. As clearly shown in Sam's story, you may both be working toward a 'normal' labour and birth when circumstances change – slowly or suddenly. Decisions will then be made by your health professional in the interest of your partner and baby. Your partner may need an assisted delivery or a caesarean.

Assisted delivery

For a number of reasons, the last stage of the birth may raise concerns. These concerns relate to the distress of your partner or the baby, so a decision may be made that your partner needs help in the final part of the process. This help is usually in the form of 'pulling' the baby through the birth canal. The doctor will use either forceps or a ventouse.

The *ventouse* is a suction cap that fits on the baby's head. As Steve said, it looks like the plumber's instrument used to clear blocked drains. *Forceps* are metal spoons. They look like a type of salad server. Both instruments allow the doctor to gently guide the baby out while your partner pushes. They are regarded as safe but may leave some bruising on the baby's head. This should disappear in the first few weeks after the birth. The ventouse may also leave the baby with a cone-shaped head for a few days.

Caesarean

A caesarean is an operation that results in the baby being taken out through the stomach. It can be a planned procedure, as described by Tom, or unplanned, as was the case with Sam and his partner.

If planned, you will have received information from your doctor regarding the reason, the timing and the actual procedure.

If the decision to deliver your baby by caesarean occurs as the result of complications, you might not be able to witness the birth.

Usually a decision is made during labour, based on the progress or wellbeing of your baby, and there will be an opportunity to discuss what is happening with your doctor. In this case you will more than likely be able to accompany your partner into theatre. This is known as a non-emergency caesarean, and your partner will be given an *epidural anaesthetic* that allows her to be awake during the procedure.

Occasionally, however, the decision to carry out a caesarean has to be made quickly. It then becomes an emergency procedure, which does not allow time for discussion or even much explanation. Your partner will be quickly taken to theatre and will most likely be given a *general anaesthetic*. She will be unconscious during the operation, and you will not be allowed to accompany her.

As with any surgical procedure, there are risks associated with a caesarean. Complications are not common, but your partner will have to go through a recovery phase. As Tom recalled, it took time for his partner to get over the operation, and her stay in hospital was extended.

You're a dad!

The time has come. Your baby has entered the world and you are a father.

> 'It's difficult to explain how I felt when I saw my baby. It was like nothing I've felt before. I just felt this rush of emotion. It was love at first sight. I just wanted to hold her and make sure she was real.'
>
> Richard, 35

> 'It was unreal. I was no longer tired. It was like I'd been given a shot of adrenaline. Nothing else mattered. This was my son.'
>
> James, 33

Your baby will be checked out, and if everything is okay, she will be given to you and your partner. These are your first moments as a family.

How will they check your baby?

Within the first minute of birth, your baby will be assessed and given an Apgar score. The staff at the hospital or birthing centre will check your baby's overall condition to identify whether she requires immediate medical assistance. They will check her heart rate, respiratory effort, muscle tone, reflexes and colour. Your baby receives a score of 0, 1 or 2 in each of the five areas. A score of 7 to 10 indicates that the baby is in good condition. Most babies don't receive a score of 10 on the first test. A second test is done five minutes later, and for most babies their score increases. As mentioned, this is a 'quick test' to determine whether immediate help is required. A more thorough examination of your baby will occur during the next 24 hours.

What if your baby needs extra help?

Some babies do need extra help after the birth.

If your baby was premature (born before 37 weeks) or experienced problems during the birth, she may require time in the *Special Care Nursery*. The main purpose of this unit is to closely monitor the progress of your baby and provide any medical treatment required.

A common reason for babies spending time in this nursery is *jaundice*. If your baby has jaundice, her skin will have a yellow tinge. This is common in newborn babies, particularly if they are premature. It is the result of an immature liver trying to break down excess red blood cells that are no longer required. In most cases, babies receive a clean bill of health after a few days. They may spend some time 'sunbaking' under an ultraviolet light. In a small number of cases, jaundice may require longer monitoring, but further medical intervention is rare.

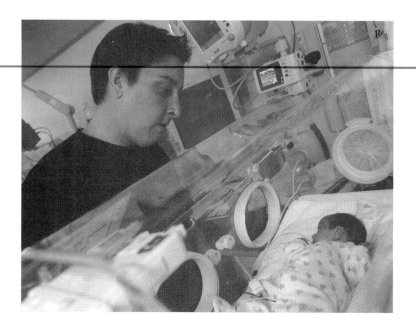

You can accompany your baby to the Special Care Nursery, and you should be encouraged to have plenty of physical contact with your baby while she is there, unless there is a medical reason not to. Most health professionals recognise the benefits of parents' physical contact for premature and sick babies.

If your baby's condition is serious or life-threatening, it may be necessary for her to be placed in a *Neonatal Intensive Care Unit*. These are not available in all hospitals and she may need to be transferred to another location. It is doubtful that your partner will be in any condition to travel, but you should be encouraged to accompany your baby. This can be a daunting experience for any parent, but your baby will be receiving the help she needs; the expertise of the staff and the equipment available can improve the outcomes for your baby.

Your presence and, if possible, physical contact can make a difference.

'What happened following the birth was pretty dramatic. I knew something was wrong but didn't know what. They rushed our baby out of the room and seemed really concerned. A nurse returned and said our baby had heart problems. They weren't sure what exactly was wrong but it was serious. They were going to fly her to another hospital that had a special unit. They asked me if I wanted to go with the baby, and after checking with my partner, I grabbed the chance.

I didn't find out much on the flight and I was told they wouldn't know more until tests were done. In the special unit, it was scary seeing my tiny baby hooked up to all those machines. She was there for two weeks and I stayed in accommodation at the hospital. Most of the time, I sat beside the cot talking to her and gently touching her. I went through stages of fear and even despair in the first few days, not knowing if she would survive. At last things improved, and my partner joined us after four days. We were told that an operation might be necessary and that her condition would be monitored over the next few months before any decision was made. It hasn't been easy, but the medication has worked and any decision about an operation has been delayed until she is at least two. I know I will always regard her as a miracle and those early days have resulted in a special bond between us.'

David, 36

All parents hope for a healthy baby, but things can go wrong. The advances in treatment and the incredible expertise of health professionals continue to improve the outcomes for seriously ill babies. The importance of parents in any treatment is now also recognised and valued.

Summary

★ Labour and birth is a time of anxiety, excitement – and miracles.

★ During the first and second stages of labour, the birth of your child and immediately after the birth, there are plenty of ways you can be involved.

★ Complications such as emergency caesareans, assisted deliveries, jaundice and premature births can occur, so it pays to be informed.

★ Physical contact with parents is important for all babies, including premature or sick babies.

6 Coming home – the first six weeks

The congratulatory calls have stopped, and the experts have begun to emerge (watch out for the gratuitous advice – you will have to get used to this!). The flowers are beginning to wilt. And the late-night suburban serenity is being broken by a baby demanding to be fed.

What an experience bringing a child home can be! You suddenly realise that the baby is yours, and that there is an important new person around the house needing care and attention. There is also another person to interact with, to hold, cuddle and love, and someone who can provoke pride, pleasure,

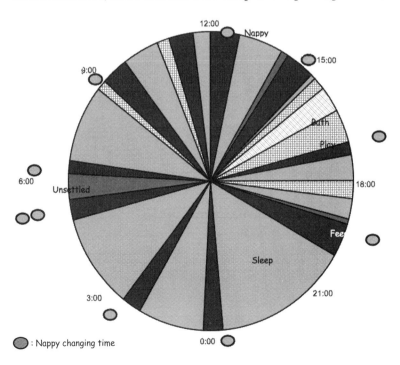

: Nappy changing time

fascination and satisfaction. For many of us this is a new type of experience. The baby becomes the focus of our lives, and our needs become quite secondary.

Some fathers find it useful to monitor the baby's patterns. A new dad, Damian, even plotted his baby's life on a graph! (See p. 115)

In this chapter, we focus on the following:

★ fathers' feelings and responses to coming home with a baby

★ the type of involvement possible for you at this stage, including taking full responsibility for your new baby

★ whether babies respond differently to mothers and fathers

★ the importance of teamwork

★ Postnatal depression in mothers – and fathers.

Fathers' feelings and responses to baby coming home

First, let's hear from a few fathers who have been through this experience.

> 'We have twins – so I expect it happened at twice the pace! I still have the most vivid memories of arriving home and being hit by the fact that these were our babies. We now had the sole responsibility for them. The hospital just packed us off – standard routine, nothing special, out the

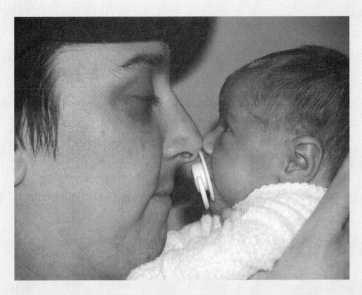

door, an expectation that you would cope. It was like we should have known what to do. Were we prepared for this? I can't remember any course that told you about the first few days and weeks, or specifically what to expect when you arrived home. We had prepared the nursery, we had prepared for the birth, but as for preparing for having the responsibility for two new babies at home alone – nothing! One thing I'm glad about is that I was there. I had taken leave from my work for a week. I had made the decision to take leave then rather than when Maryanne was in hospital. I am glad I did.'

Peter, 38

These comments from Peter emphasise the importance of getting involved from the start and sharing these experiences as a couple.

'I was working part-time when Sarah came home, so I was around every morning. I worked from twelve to six. Like

Peter, I was blown away by the experience. I had not been able to imagine what it would be like. This small person – so dependent, such a mystery. What was she thinking? What was she feeling? What did she want? Were we doing the right thing? From my mother's perspective, it seemed we weren't! She had other ideas about what we should be doing in terms of sleep and feeding – her way was certainly the best!'

James, 29

'My family was great. They weren't intrusive, they were very supportive. They cooked us several meals, dropped by every now and then, and phoned a lot. Eventually, we had to get them to stop phoning quite as much. It became annoying because it was waking up Sam – and us as well when we were trying to cat-nap. One thing I do remember consulting them on was how to do the bathing. We read about it in the books and we figured we were doing okay, but Sam cried all the time – he didn't seem to like it at all. In the end we had a couple of communal baths. No, not all in together – all of us standing around watching my mum and dad bathing Sam. Seeing this, we figured we were doing very well! What we needed was a little reassurance – we needed to be confident we were doing the right thing.'

John, 31

What a good idea, a communal bath! The best part about this story is the power of observational learning – watching someone do a task that you are uncertain about. The grandparents provided the necessary reassurance and John and his partner were then able to bath their baby with much more confidence.

'I must say, I was a bit anxious too because Julie didn't seem very confident to me. I found this a surprise as she had always been super confident in all aspects of her life. I found it hard to tell her this or to discuss it openly to check on how she felt. I was going on what I saw. Julie asked her mother lots of questions, but all of this was so far back in her mother's past she couldn't remember. I am not sure how we worked through it – I think Julie must have talked to her friends. She seemed to make lots of phone calls in the first few days, but then we worked through things, and by the third day she seemed to be on top of it all.'

Darren, 33

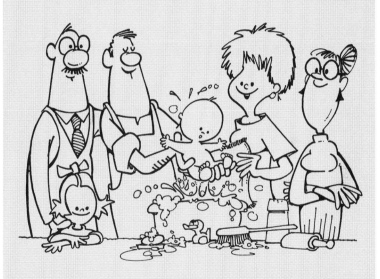

This comes as a surprise to a lot of new fathers and mothers. Society has high expectations for new mothers: that they will know all about babies, that they will have all the necessary skills – that caring for a newborn will come naturally to them. The reality is that while the emotional connection is there for mothers and fathers, competent care of a newborn benefits from knowledge, practice and support.

'I hadn't expected to be around when we brought our baby home. It was a very demanding time at work – there was so much happening and I had several deadlines looming. But things didn't go as planned with the birth – she was nine weeks premature. Hariette was in a humidicrib with wires and cords going everywhere. She also got a lot of attention from doctors and nurses. This really freaked me out, so much so that work was not even on the radar screen. I was at the hospital as much as I could be. Things improved, but it seemed like an eternity before they did. Being around at home in the first few weeks was what I needed to do, for myself, for Hariette and for Melissa. Hariette took some time before she was a reasonable weight to come home. And Melissa had considerable difficulty in breastfeeding. Being there to give her support and encouragement was very important at that stage.'

Philip, 24

'I was warned about the lack of sleep when you have a new baby, but it still turned me inside out. You know, when there was just the two of us we were night owls. We partied and it was nothing to get only a few hours' sleep between Friday and Monday. The difference was that we knew we could at some time crash and catch up. Not true with a baby. For the first week I made the effort to get up with Sue when she did the night feeds. It really got to me in the second week. I started pretending that I didn't hear Sue get up. She let me sleep. When I went back to work I told Sue I needed my sleep as I had to work. She didn't say anything. The truth was I found it easier to go to work even with broken sleep. Tom was not good at night and it came to a point where I felt so bloody guilty about leaving all the night stuff to Sue that I started getting up. She really appreciated the help. There were times when both of us would have gladly taken Tom and put him on the neighbour's doorstep – I mean they were a nice family. At the time, you think it is never going to end, but it does. He actually increased his night sleep to five hours after about seven weeks – it seemed like ten years at the time. Then, at about three months, he started again – every two hours. I reckon he was just giving us time to recoup.'

Kevin, 26

For many fathers the increased emotional and physical demands (e.g. due to having a premature baby or due to disrupted sleep) present significant challenges to their own wellbeing, their relationship with their partner and their capacity to maintain their paid work commitments. While it is true that nothing lasts forever and that things can change quickly, an option to consider here (and to plan for) is to take leave from work or reduce your work commitments for two to four weeks. You and your baby will certainly be happier for this!

'Yes, we needed some reassurance as well. In the end we realised we were doing fine. We had an Early Childhood Nurse come to our house and visit us to check that things were going okay. When this was arranged, I thought it was intrusive. I was very apprehensive: I thought they might have been checking on us to see if we were competent parents – a kind of big brother parenting audit. They didn't offer appointments out of regular hours so I took time off work to be there. The nurse obviously didn't expect me to be there as she directed most of her questions and conversation to Annette. But I took the same approach as I had done at the hospital. I introduced myself, remembered her name and thought about her as being part of our team – at least for the time she was there. I took the opportunity to ask some questions of my own. I think she was surprised when I asked her about Kate's nappy rash. It was a very comforting experience. We felt much better about how we were doing and it provided us with the opportunity to ask questions that we wondered about, but didn't know who to ask. I felt it was more equal and relaxed in our home. This service should be offered to all first-time parents, and especially to first-time fathers.'

Nathan, 35

'Suzanne went to an Early Childhood Centre with Rebecca. I didn't go. I didn't realise it was an option. I figured it was for mothers and babies. This wasn't an entirely happy experience for us. Rebecca got a positive score card except that the nurse said she was being overfed. We thought this was strange as we didn't think a breastfed baby could be overfed. We didn't take any notice and continued to do what we were doing. I also remember that Suzanne came back with some new ideas about sleeping. I thought we had figured this out and had agreed that what we were doing was the best for Rebecca. We spent a few days working through our different ideas again and sorting things out. I think this is something you have to be careful of – the extent to which you allow outside experts to influence you and how this works itself out in your relationship with your partner. We nearly came to blows about this.'

John, 25

The issues raised by Nathan and John above are critical to think about. Having community support, especially in facilitating the healthy development of a newborn, is important. Health professionals are able to identify potential health problems with babies early on and thus prevent more serious health issues. The involvement of these professionals can present issues for some fathers as they may feel that they are not included, or that they are excluded on the assumption they are not important. When mothers are responding to advice from 'outside', there is also the potential for conflict in the relationship. An option here is to do what Nathan did – be confident and assertive and get involved. Importantly, ask questions and seek information.

The message from these fathers is that bringing home a new baby can be a bit of a shock. Not bringing your baby home immediately, say because of health issues or because he was born prematurely, can be an even bigger shock. There are feelings of uncertainty, there is a need for reassurance and, most importantly, there is good reason to be around to share the experience, whether it is at home or in the hospital. Teamwork is critical at this stage – working with your partner and also including others (such as an Early Childhood Nurse and other family members) to support you when needed. Sometimes you may need a coach or confidant. You could find it helpful to have someone to talk to about what is going on and what you are experiencing and feeling. A good friend who is also a father (this could be your own father) is often a good source of advice and support.

What can you do?

- Take time off work to be at home during the first week or two when your baby comes home.
- If you have a visit from an Early Childhood Nurse or an appointment at an Early Childhood Centre, try to be there with your partner. Be involved in making the appointment so that you can find a time that fits in with your work.
- Think of yourself as part of the team – get involved and ask questions when you interact with health professionals.
- Remember that your relationship with your partner is important – say and do things that tell her you love and value her as a partner and a mother.
- Write a summary of your experiences in your parenting diary and share these with a friend who is a new dad or about to become a dad.
- Consider the following advice from Sarah Macdonald – this applies to fathers as well as mothers.

FASCINATING FACTS ABOUT PARENTING

In a response to an article in the *Sydney Morning Herald* on 22 July 2004 which suggested that 'Parents lack the skills to raise children and need more help', Sarah Macdonald, talking from a personal perspective, provided some reassurance for new parents. Her message was that caring for your first baby is tough, but millions have managed to do it. In her words:

'When a midwife saw my husband and I nervously delay taking our baby into the world of the unknown she came in for a valuable chat. She told us she felt the modern parents who strictly follow books and over-analyse our babies run the risk of raising potentially neurotic children. She told us not to worry too much, saying: "After all, we had no idea what we were doing either, no-one does at first". I took her advice to heart and tried to follow my instinct, my baby and what worked, while staying open-minded to the research, philosophies and plethora of information coming my way. And I was comforted on the few times I did call in the professionals, to find they were often as dumbfounded as I… Mothers' groups, baby health care clinics, parenting classes and playgroups all normalise our confusion, give valuable support and provide an essential outlet to indulge our obsessions. I recommend to all parents, experienced or otherwise, use them.'

Sarah Macdonald, 'Fascinating experiences as a parent',
Sydney Morning Herald, 23 July 2004

What type of involvement is possible for dads?

Although the traditional view has been that mothers are more competent than fathers, and indeed that they might even have a biological advantage over fathers in having the skills and sensitivity to care for a newborn baby, not all mothers agree. When faced with the hard realities of caring for a newborn baby, many mothers experience difficulties and find that they have not much more idea than their partners. Caring for a newborn involves a diversity of learned skills, and while on average women are more likely to learn these skills as they grow up (e.g. by having had more prior experience in caring for children), men can catch up very quickly, especially when they have their own child.

'I agree. I found that when we arrived home we both floundered for the first day or so. The clear memory I have is that Janice had no more skills than I had. She had some theories, some ideas about what to do, but in practice we were not much different. We both had to learn and, importantly, we both had to tune in to our baby. What was really critical was to learn first to focus on our baby – to accept that her needs should be met first – and to try to understand our baby. I figured the only thing I couldn't do was breastfeed. Even so, I often sat with them during the feeds and I took over as soon as the feed was finished.'

William, 29

'It is the experience that counts, being there, having to make the decision, practising, changing nappies, bathing, settling – it's a learning journey. We all have our own idiosyncrasies. I am not a great singer, but I loved singing to Christina. When she was upset, I would cuddle her and sing. I am not sure it always soothed her, but she knew I cared and that I was trying to fix things for her. And it was good for me. I enjoyed it. As they say in the management books – it was a win, win, win!'

Steven, 41

'I'm not sure I agree with you that men can be just as good at this as women can. Kerryn is a natural. She always knows what Brendon needs – she always knows what is wrong. She just has that knack that I don't seem to have. She always seemed to be commenting on what I did as well. I was fine with this up to a point, but I must say, I enjoyed the times Kerryn went out and left me with Brendon – I could do things my way then.'

Albert, 36

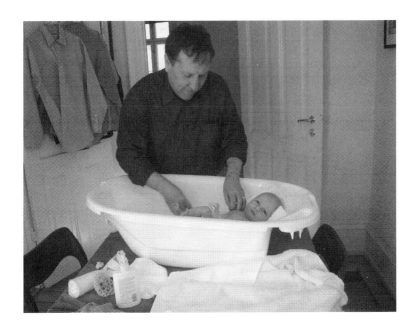

What can be learned from these comments and from the research is that given the opportunity and experience, fathers can be just as competent at childcare as mothers. In one research study, mothers and fathers were observed interacting with their newborns: the fathers were as involved with the newborns as the mothers, and equally nurturing (e.g. in touching, looking at, kissing and talking to their babies). If bottle-feeding, fathers were equally likely to detect and respond appropriately to the cues of their baby, such as sucking, burping and coughing, and just as successful (as measured by the amount of milk consumed by the infant).

'I don't believe in a maternal instinct. It's all rubbish. If a person wants to – if a man wants to – he can do it just as well. Obviously he can't breastfeed, but he can do everything else.'

Michael, 41

'I like to cuddle my baby. Maybe there is a paternal instinct. That seems to strike a responsive chord with me. I like to cuddle babies. My baby responds to smiles, responds to the sound of my voice.'

Randell, 35

There seems no reason why fathers can't become involved in every aspect of caring for a baby: soothing and comforting, nappy changing, dressing and bathing, and singing! What most fathers need (as do mothers) is the relevant information and practice – some on-the-job learning – just as for so many other skills we acquire in our lives. In terms of connecting with your baby, the rewards for becoming involved in this way are enormous. From the very beginning you can start to build the foundation for your lifelong relationship. Your baby will also appreciate getting to know you – and the variety they experience when at least two people are providing care for them, in slightly different ways; they certainly notice the difference in voices.

It is also true that some of us (both fathers and mothers) cope 'better' with the demands of childcare than others – and some of us have more demanding babies than others. We also have our on and off days, when we are in better or worse moods. We can experience difficulties in keeping up with the changing fashions in infant care or worry about whether we are being 'good enough' parents. We all want to be the best parents we can, and one way for fathers to become more skilful and knowledgeable about the needs of their baby is to be the sole caregiver at regular times during the week.

Have a go on your own!

As anyone who has constant responsibility for the care of young babies and children knows, having someone to share this with, to support you and to take over at different times is something to value and look forward to. This is a key part of working together as a team. Fathers who spend time alone with their babies all say that the relationship improves dramatically – they say they really get to know their baby. It is not simply the extra time that is important, but how this time is spent. Having the sole responsibility helps you to develop your own special relationship and your own way of doing tasks and organising things. It also allows you to handle the special, sensitive times when your baby needs attention (e.g. when he is crying when you know he should be asleep). Importantly too, it helps you to build your self-confidence as a father.

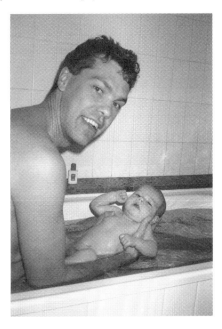

FASCINATING FACTS ABOUT FATHERS

Research shows that, on average, few fathers spend a lot of time alone with their children, yet those who do report that doing this leads to a significantly improved relationship – based in part on their improved understanding of their children and the connection established by sharing activities together.

Keep in mind, too, that babies have different temperaments. Infants vary considerably in how 'easy' or 'difficult' they are. There is little you can do about this, at least in the first few months. *Easy babies* are sometimes classified as those who always seem to be in a good mood, who go to sleep easily, and who are regular and predictable (well, not 100 per cent of the time) and very responsive to adults. *Difficult babies* are seen as those who are frequently irritable and cry a lot, and have more difficulty sleeping and settling. Other babies – such as those who are *slow to warm up* – often seem to be shy and less responsive to new situations, and, at times, less active. Parents sometimes have one who is easy, one who is difficult and one who is a mixture of both (they couldn't really be classified using this system).

What can you do?

- Keep your focus on your baby so that you learn about your baby's patterns. Be alert to and curious about your baby. All babies are different: they have different temperaments, different sleeping patterns and different needs for social interaction.
- *You have the opportunity to get involved in every aspect, so be prepared to learn and try things out for yourself. Don't stand back; take the initiative – be assertive when you need to.* One father we came across used to demand his own special bonding times on the weekends. He figured that his partner had more than her share during the week!
- Spend some time alone with your infant. This is good for your connection with your child and it provides some free time for your partner. It is a key aspect of teamwork at this stage.

Do babies respond differently to mothers and fathers?

One of the strongest held beliefs about parenting has been that the mother–infant relationship is unique, that the infant becomes attached to the mother, and that this mother–infant attachment is necessary in the short-term (e.g. for emotional and social development) and in the long-term (e.g. for their ability to form deep relationships with other people). However, research shows that security of attachment to both mother and father is linked to positive outcomes for children. It pays off in the long run if you are able to establish this type of relationship with your child. In the words of Professor Bryanne Barnett, 'How parents look at and talk to their baby is crucial to a child's development. A baby needs to see in the carer's face that it is loved and lovable. The relationship with carers, established in that first year, is the foundation relationship that sets up patterns for life.'

Although there is probably something special about a child's relationship with its caregivers, especially because of the unconditional nature of the love provided, and the sensitivity and responsiveness, this is not unique to the mother–child relationship. In an interesting twist, there are some who argue that there is something special or essential about fathers and their relationships with their children, especially with their sons. The balance of research, however, does not support this proposition.

Infants from around six months of age seek to be close to both their mothers and their fathers, protesting when they leave them, and looking to them for security and comfort (especially when they are distressed or uncertain); and they are glad to see them after a period of separation. We know as fathers that we have these kinds of experiences with our infants. They are attached to us as well. It depends on our sensitivity and responsiveness to their needs, and on the sheer quantity and nature of the time we share with them.

Several studies indicate that infants with more responsive parents are more secure, more sociable and more independent. Also, parental responsiveness (within reason) is relevant throughout the age range. Older children are more likely to be easier to manage too if you know how and when to respond sensitively and appropriately. Being engaged will allow you to feel more confident and competent as a parent as well; you will have more celebrations as a father, and you'll have a more enjoyable fatherhood experience. And research also shows that being confident and competent as a parent is critical for child outcomes. What fathers do does matter to their children!

FASCINATING FACTS ABOUT FATHERS

As Michael Lamb, who is widely recognised as the pre-eminent authority on fatherhood, has reported, 'The characteristics of individual fathers – such as their masculinity, intellect, or personality – are less influential in how children turn out than is the quality of the relationship a father has with his children.' Getting and staying connected with your child is critical.

Two other things to keep in mind here are that fathers are people too and that fathers matter! First, as a father you have your own moods and personality, and your children will respond differently to you because of this. Indeed, one of Graeme's children displayed a determined preference to have him change her dirty nappies! The bottom line here is that you need to focus on your child – on his needs and on his best interests.

FASCINATING FACTS ABOUT FATHERS

- Parents – both fathers and mothers – cope with the demands of a new baby better when they get on well as a couple.
- Fathers, on average, have been found to have the same kind of emotional arousal in response to their newborn babies as mothers do – they are excited, fascinated and overwhelmed, and feel a strong sense of love for them, sometimes described as a 'strong bond'.
- Babies usually 'bond' just as easily with fathers as with mothers.
- Fathers can be just as skilful at caring for babies as mothers.

What can you do?

- Be active and involved in all aspects of caring for your child, as a way of understanding your child – her/his needs, daily patterns and moods.
- Be persistent in finding your space and developing your relationship with your baby.
- Be consistent in being available, in responding and in being a key member of the team.
- Look for ways to build a sense of fairness or equity into sharing the pleasures and the day-to-day tasks of parenting (some of which are not always the most pleasurable).

Why is teamwork so important?

The absence of conflict and hostility in a family is one of the most consistent predictors of positive outcomes for children. Having a good relationship and getting on with the mother of your child is one of your major responsibilities. It is the team that counts!

We also know that having a good quality, supportive relationship helps promote our own wellbeing. Indeed, it can be a critical buffer to the other stresses we experience in life. Coming home to a supportive, caring partner, for example, can help us cope with pressures in the workplace. And from your partner's perspective, having a caring, supportive partner who will come home and change the dynamic of a stressful day with baby helps her to develop resilience and a renewed capacity to be caring and responsive to baby.

Having a baby, but particularly having a first baby, can be one of the most stressful events a couple will experience. This is when teamwork really needs to kick in. As we indicated in Chapter 1, it's a good idea to consider teamwork from several perspectives, including the sharing of tasks, caring for each other and having a strong relationship.

Fundamentally, it is the nature of your relationship with your partner that matters most. It is so easy, though, to let this aspect of teamwork slip by unnoticed. During research in the workplace, Graeme found it is very common for fathers to realise (once their children are older) that the priority they gave to their relationship decreased in an unintended way once they had children. This process of decline often began when they had their first baby.

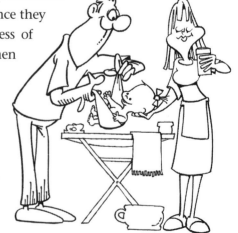

The 'busyness' of having a baby and coping with life simply meant that time was not put into their relationship. Critically, too, they found that the tension and conflict in their relationships increased – there was more to have disagreements about. Some also found that the love and intimacy they shared decreased; but many fathers had a strong desire to improve their relationships.

What matters most in relationships? It is sharing activities, spending time together, sharing the little things that matter at the end of the day, having a caring, supportive person to talk to, and being positive in your interactions (i.e. affirming the other person). Relationships are more likely to continue if the ratio of positives to negatives is in the range of 5 to 1.

So what are the danger signs? And what have other fathers found useful in improving their relationships?

'We let things drift along. I was quite happy for Sarah to take the major responsibility for caring for Rebecca; I had my work and my interests. Sure I was helpful, but I didn't ever think of it as a team activity, nor of the need for team building. Funny that, as I am the person responsible for building executive teams in my organisation. I go to great lengths to ensure that their relationships are sustained and every now and then put in place relationship renewal processes – we call them corporate retreats. Somehow, I didn't even see the connection with having a baby. Luckily for everyone, I realised this after about six months. I could see that things weren't going well: there was tension and there was resentment. When someone pointed out the teamwork analogy, it all clicked. We do more things together now – both with the baby and without her. I took over responsibility for organising our social connections – our personal retreats – and I organised my parents to look after Rebecca. Many of these were surprises for Sarah. Sarah also got into the

> spirit of our new relationship and sprung a few surprises as well – but they are personal!'
>
> John, 39

Some fathers find that things don't go as smoothly as they had anticipated and they experience some distance and tension in their relationships. For some this is linked to their partner having difficulties in adjusting to the demands of a baby.

What about postnatal depression in mothers – and fathers?

> 'I remember how great it was to have Sue and Ben at home. Sue was over the moon – she seemed so happy. The first two weeks were a bit of a blur. The broken sleep didn't seem to worry Sue. She was thriving on being a mum and I was amazed at how happy she looked. I was trying to help but she wanted to do most of the baby stuff herself. It was as if she couldn't get enough of holding and caring for Ben.
>
> I went back to work after two weeks and I started to see a change in Sue. I would come home to find her upset and she would talk about how Ben had cried for most of the day. This was a different Sue. Everything seemed so difficult for her and she was so tense. I started ringing home regularly during the day and she always complained that she couldn't settle Ben. She would give me Ben as soon as I walked in the door and say "It's your turn". I did as much as I could but it never seemed to be enough – or I wasn't doing it right.

One night I came home to find Sue in the garage crying. As soon as she saw me, she started screaming that she couldn't cope with Ben's crying. I took her inside and tried to calm her down. She kept talking about how hard it was being home all day with Ben. I got scared about what was happening to Sue and suggested we talk to our doctor. She finally agreed and we went the next day. The doctor said Sue was suffering from postnatal depression and referred her to a social worker.

Sue started going to a group and it seemed to help a bit. I still didn't know what I should do and it got so that I dreaded coming home. I felt bloody useless and all I wanted was the old Sue back. I finally rang the social worker and asked what I should do. She explained that Sue was feeling overwhelmed by being a mum and was feeling guilty that she couldn't cope. She gave me some ideas on how to help. It took a while, but Sue improved. I think they should include dads in these groups they run. What affects Sue affects me, and it would have been easier if I had known what was happening from the beginning.'

Nathan, 31

The whole area of postnatal depression is a minefield. Even estimates of incidence talk of anything from 10 to 25 per cent of women experiencing depression. From Tony's experience it appears that, as with most depression, it is rarely acknowledged that postnatal depression can vary from mild to severe. The causes also vary, and can include previous conditions and experiences of the mother; experiences of trauma, such as abuse; birth experiences; the baby's temperament; available support; and the mum's expectations. Tony's experience also suggests that dads are too often left out of any intervention – postnatal depression groups are usually run for women during the day, with at most a 'meeting' with partners. Big mistake! As Nathan said, what happens to the mother affects all members of the new family, including Dad. If services don't include the father, they risk reducing the support available to the mother, and this could prolong the depression and increase its impact. Dads can provide understanding, reassurance, and a range of practical and emotional supports that can help the family through this difficult time.

Dads can also experience depression following the birth of their baby. I guess Tony's take on this is similar – severity and causes vary. His experience suggests, too, that dads are less likely to have their depression diagnosed; less likely to seek or receive help; and more likely to adopt behaviours that involve escape, denial and use of alcohol.

'I was looking forward to having a baby but something happened after Brendan had been home a few weeks. I found it hard to concentrate at work and I became really anxious that something was going to happen to Brendan. I had no reason to worry, as he seemed to be thriving – but I did worry. Every little task just seemed so difficult. I couldn't settle him and he seemed to cry every time I picked him up. I backed off from caring for him and started spending more time at work. This didn't help as I wasn't interested in what I was doing. The only time I felt okay was when I'd had a few drinks. Karen was pretty tolerant but my boss wasn't. He made it clear that my work wasn't up to scratch and put me on notice that if things didn't improve he would have to act. I didn't know what was happening, but it scared me. I told Karen about work and she told me I

> had better do something as she was sick and tired of how I was at home. I finally agreed to talk to our doctor and he told me I had depression. It was a relief to have someone explain what was happening. I went to counselling and came to realise that I had had similar episodes at earlier stages of my life. I had suffered without saying anything and again never really understood what was happening. I started to understand that the life change of having a baby had triggered my depression. It took time but I got back to enjoying being a dad – and I kept my job.'
>
> Andrew, 31

Services that focus only on mother and baby risk excluding an important member of the family – the father. Including Dad provides opportunities to strengthen the family and helps identify problems that will respond to early intervention.

What can you do if your partner is depressed?

It is important that you regularly check with your partner about how she is feeling. Don't assume that because she is a woman she will be a 'supermum' at all times. Your involvement in daily care activities can help take the pressure off, but if you are concerned, you need to recommend that you both talk to your local doctor – and be open and honest in your communication.

Your partner may resist help at first, feeling that she 'should be able to cope'. Don't give up. If she agrees to seek help, be involved. Remember that what affects your partner will affect you – and more importantly, your understanding of what's happening. Having information about what you can do to help *can make a difference*.

Summary

★ Coming home with your baby can be an absolute pleasure – one of the true highs of your life – and it can also be overwhelming.

★ Contrary to a common assumption from previous generations, fathers and mothers are equally competent as caregivers. And like mothers, some fathers readily warm to this involvement and responsibility, and some don't.

★ Having a go on your own is one of the ways you can develop the confidence to craft your own special relationship with your child.

★ Equally important is being part of the team – working together to make this sometimes difficult time work for everyone. No-one is built to care for children 24/7 on their own!

★ If either you or your partner is depressed following the birth of your child, seek help – together.

★ And don't forget your relationship – children tend to respond better when you have a good relationship with your partner.

7 What babies need

In your journey as a parent there will be challenges – challenges as an individual, as a partner and, of course, as a father. In considering these challenges, it is important to keep in mind that parenting *is about children*.

In this chapter we discuss what babies need on their journey to a happy childhood and how parents can support their development. We will accompany babies through the first six months of life and listen to their 'stories' as they reflect on their travels from birth. The stories will be based on our experience and what research tells us about this time in their lives. We will also discuss how parents can work together in providing the care that ensures the best possible start to this incredible journey.

Let's imagine a group of six-month-old babies reflecting on their journeys from birth. How will they adapt to their new life? How will they make sense of it all? What do they need?

Babies' thoughts on the big journey

This is what Jessica, Joel, Tom, Julie, Brendon and Stephanie have to say.

'It was a bit shaky at first. I think all babies should be given an instruction book on how to survive new parents. I knew from the start that Dad and Mum wanted to be the best parents in the world. What they seemed to lack was experience in knowing what I needed and how to provide it. My needs were pretty basic in those early days. I needed food, somewhere comfortable to sleep and lots of cuddles.

How could I let Dad and Mum know what I wanted? I tried talking to them, but all that came out of my mouth was "waaaah".

I asked for food, and out came "waaaah". I asked for cuddles – same thing – "waaaah". I tried changing the tone. I varied the number of "waaaahs".

Whenever I talked they got worried looks on their faces – but they did pick me up. Right – "waaaah" works. I knew then that given time we would get to know each other.'

Jessica, 6 months

'I remember Mum and Dad discussing breastfeeding even before I was born. They read books and went to classes. The message was constant – "Breast is best". It made sense to me – no preparation time, easy to transport, attractive containers, and the cat couldn't get it.

I thought it would be so easy. When I was hungry, just put me on the nipple. Boy was I wrong! Mum went through a pretty rough time learning to feed me. She had to hold me in a certain position and I took some time adjusting. The nurses in the hospital helped, but when we got home it was as if we had to start all over again.

We all went to see the Child and Family Health Nurse for a bit of help. It started to work and I got really good at getting enough to eat.

I think parents need to be supported when they start breastfeeding. They also need to be told the truth: it can be difficult at first.

Dad needed to be told that he would find it stressful to see Mum and I upset when we ran into problems. His support was so important.'

Joel, 6 months

'I don't like to talk too much about my bodily functions, but it seemed like a big deal for Mum and Dad. At first they got excited if I did something and would smile a lot as they cleaned me up – so I kept doing it, as often as possible. My favourite was doing it as soon as they changed me. No smiles then – just a funny grin.

Dad made the mistake of putting his hand down my nappy to check if I'd done anything. He only did it the once. From then on he would hold me up and smell me.

The thing I remember most was how Dad would talk to me and blow bubbles on my tummy when he changed me. It was never boring. It was a great way to get to know each other. It also showed me he cared.'

Tom, 6 months

'I couldn't believe it. I'd only been born a couple of days and they stuck me in 2 centimetres of tepid water. What had I done wrong? I let them know I wasn't impressed in no uncertain terms. Would you believe it, they did it again when I got home – and they continued doing it nearly every day.

They seemed surprised – even distressed – that I didn't like lying in cold water covered with this soapy stuff.

I remember Dad muttering about how embarrassing it

was to have a child who hated water when we lived near the ocean. Hey, make the water warm and maybe I'll stop crying.

After talking to a number of other kids, I realised it was a common problem with new parents. They were terrified that I'd get burnt if the water was too hot. So they kept putting their elbow in to test the temperature. Of course, their elbows got more sensitive with each test and the water they finally decided on was just above polar conditions. When they took me shopping, I could spot a new parent by the blisters on their elbow!

Good old Dad came to the rescue. He suggested I have a bath with him. Made sense to me – if it burnt his bum, it would burn mine. Also, he wasn't about to sit in freezing water!

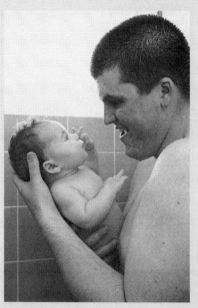

It worked well. I enjoyed my bath. Dad would wash me, then hand me over to Mum to do the drying. Good teamwork.'

Julie, 6 months

'When I was first born I slept for most of the first day. I was worn out from the birth. I think Mum and Dad thought this was going to be the norm. No way! They talk about the average baby sleeping for about sixteen hours a day in the first few weeks – well, I'm far from average.

I slept for about ten hours each day – in sessions of two hours. This was all I needed in the first six weeks. Mum and Dad got a hell of a shock. Within five days they both had this glazed look on their face.

They took me to the doctor and the baby clinic, thinking there was something wrong with me. I was studied, poked, prodded and pronounced healthy. "You have a baby that doesn't need a lot of sleep" was not the answer Dad wanted to hear.'
Brendon, 6 months

'In my case Dad and Mum tried different sleeping tactics. They wrapped me tightly, then loosely, then not at all. They tried music, rocking, walking and even driving in the car. Dad said I saw more of our neighbourhood in three weeks than he had seen in thirty years.

At about three weeks I slept for five hours straight. I woke to find Mum and Dad standing over me with a feather near my mouth. They were checking my breathing. It freaked me out and I immediately went back to my two hours.

I finally started sleeping through most of the night after a couple of months and I think that's when Mum and Dad stopped talking about adoption.'
Stephanie, 6 months

At first it can be daunting for new parents when they arrive home with their baby. The baby seems even smaller and more helpless than when she was in hospital. Where are the nurses to explain what the baby needs?

Getting to know your baby takes time and practice.

As Jessica said, her needs in the beginning were basic and involved food, physical contact and sleep. It is important to recognise that when providing the daily care you are doing more than meeting those basic needs. You are getting to know your baby – and she is getting to know you. Of course, it would make your job easier if babies could tell you clearly what they needed.

A response from you or your partner to their crying

Crying is a baby's most effective way of communicating. They cry if they are hungry, tired, uncomfortable or bored, or because they just want to be held. The bottom line is they want your attention.

As a parent, you will respond – and this is how it should be. Responding to the cries of a baby is not spoiling her. In fact, it is argued that if you respond to her cries her sense of security increases. This has been shown to assist greatly in her ability to settle by herself and develop good sleep patterns as she grows.

You want to provide whatever it is your baby needs, and you feel you have succeeded if the crying stops. At first you try the obvious – food, changing her nappy, cuddles. As you become more acquainted with your baby, you will often anticipate her needs before the crying starts and develop a greater range of responses when it does.

What we know about crying

It is common for crying to increase over the first six weeks. This means that you may have a baby who seldom cries when first born and then seems to practise and increase in frequency and volume.

You can expect your baby to cry for two to three hours a day during the first three months. This is an average figure, which means that many babies cry for longer periods. If you have a baby who is at the 'excessive' end of crying, you will want to know why. It is now thought that the amount of crying may be connected with the baby's development. Crying appears to peak as the baby adjusts to each stage of life in her new world.

Babies on the 'excessive' end of the crying scale are sometimes said to have colic. The symptoms of colic usually start at about three weeks and are often associated with feed times. Researchers and health professionals vary in their opinions on cause and treatment. Explanations range from food intolerance to an immature nervous system. The main message for parents is that colic causes an extreme form of crying, but thankfully it will end.

Crying can also indicate pain. When crying seems out of the ordinary, such as a sharp, sudden scream, check with your doctor. If the crying is accompanied by changes in behaviour, such as a lack of interest in feeding, seek advice. As a good rule of thumb, *if you are in doubt – check it out.*

How will you cope with your baby crying?

Each baby is an individual. They vary in their reactions to noise, bright lights and stimulation. You will get to know your baby's likes and dislikes as you provide daily care.

You are also an individual. How you cope with your baby crying will be influenced by *your* temperament. Of course, this also applies to your partner. Working as a team will make it easier.

Parents can get frustrated and even angry if they can't stop the crying. This is normal, but rarely discussed. If you do get angry, share those feelings with your partner. Talking about your feelings can help.

'Yes, I remember getting angry at Josh in the early weeks. I was angry that he wouldn't settle, angry because he was stopping me getting any decent sleep, and angry because no matter what I did it didn't seem to be enough. I felt lousy feeling this way towards my son, so I asked my dad if he got angry as a dad. He said, "All parents get angry with their children at some time – but you can't get angry at a little baby." I felt worse.

Later we had a reunion of our antenatal class and were talking about our experiences. I mentioned feeling angry at Josh and at first everyone just looked at me. Then some of the others started saying that they felt the same. I was surprised by how many of the mums started talking about their anger. One mum said, "I felt really bad and started questioning what type of woman I was. Women aren't supposed to feel angry at their babies." It helped to know what was happening was normal. Now Claire and I can say how we feel, and when either of us is feeling uptight, the other steps in and helps take the pressure off.'

Sean, 27

Many parents report that crying often 'peaks' in the evening. This is a vulnerable time after a day at work, and even more so after a day responding to the needs of your baby. Add to this the demands of cooking dinner and preparing baby for bed. If ever teamwork was important, it is now. Sharing the tasks will help.

The good news is that crying usually decreases from three months – but sometimes slowly.

Jessica's tips for dads on crying

'When I cry, I'm talking to you. You may not always understand what I'm saying, but please try to respond. Sometimes I will stop crying if I'm fed, cuddled or changed. At other times, neither of us will know what to do. With practice, we'll both learn what helps. These are some of the things that might help us through these potentially difficult times:

- Take me for a walk in the pram. You might like to do this on your own or take Mum with us. If nothing else, it's great family time and good exercise.

- Rock me gently. If you don't get a quick result, try taking turns with Mum. You could sing or hum softly while you hold me, too. I like that.

- Try a gentle massage. Massage can be used from the time I'm a few days old. At first, gently stroke my hands and feet and around my head and neck; as I get older, try a full body massage after my bath. It's a great time for us to connect.

- Buy me a dummy. Dummies can help to settle me down. It's up to you whether you want to try this. As I get older, I may need some help during the night finding my lost dummy. Some people think that as I get older the dummy may affect my speech development, and weaning me off my dummy may also be a challenge.

Make sure you enjoy the times when I'm not crying. This will help us through the hard stretches.'

Food, glorious food

Breast or bottle – this is a question for all new parents. Food and nutrition are critical for your baby's development, right from the moment of conception. What to feed your baby is one of the many decisions you will face. The decision you make will be based on information you receive, circumstances and, of course, choice.

Breastfeeding

Breastmilk is the 'perfect food' for a baby. It not only contains the right nutrients but also antibodies that protect your baby from diseases. Breastmilk decreases the chance of allergic reactions such as eczema, asthma and food intolerance.

Interestingly, breastmilk adjusts to your baby's needs. It has been shown that the composition of breastmilk changes with age to meet the developmental needs of babies.

Breastmilk comes at the right temperature. It is sterile and, of course, cheaper.

Common myths about breastfeeding

Myth 1 **Breastfeeding comes naturally to all women.** The truth is many women struggle in the early stages of breastfeeding. Success relates to the amount of support women have from health professionals and, most importantly, their partners.

Myth 2 **Your partner can't get pregnant while breast-feeding.** Don't rely on it – use appropriate contraceptives.

Myth 3 **Fathers become 'jealous' of the closeness between mother and baby during breastfeeding.** Wrong! The vast majority of fathers support breastfeeding if given the correct information.

Joel's tips for dads on breastfeeding

'Discuss feeding options with Mum before I'm born. Remember that with breastfeeding, your support is important.

If difficulties arise, encourage Mum to seek advice and support. I've been told by other kids that this is available from health professionals and the Australian Breastfeeding Association (ABA). Try to be there with Mum.

When I come home, be involved by taking me to the food source – Mum will particularly appreciate this during the night. Become part of the ritual by bringing Mum a nice cup of tea or a glass of milk, and burping and changing me after the feed.'

Supplementary feeds while breastfeeding

Supplementary feeding refers to the use of a bottle as well as the breast to feed your baby. The bottle may contain expressed breastmilk or formula. There are a number of reasons for the use of supplementary feeds, including mum returning to work, as a back-up if mum is to be away from the baby for a time, and as preparation for weaning before baby is able to use a cup.

Bottle-feeding

Circumstances or choice may mean you decide on bottle-feeding. Although there are many advantages in breastfeeding, parents should not feel guilty, or be made to feel guilty, for choosing to bottle-feed their babies.

Tony: In my role as a psychologist, I would regularly be invited to give talks to a local branch of the Nursing Mothers Association (now called the ABA). The topics related to stages of child development, from birth to the beginning of school. One evening I was asked if I supported breastfeeding in my work with new parents. I made it clear that I did support breastfeeding, but added that I had also seen the impact on women who were unable to breastfeed, or chose not to. I argued that guilt achieved nothing but negative results for parents. I encouraged the group to advocate for improved support services for parents who wanted to breastfeed, but also asked that they support all parents, regardless of their feeding choice.

At the end of my talk I was approached by a woman who wanted to thank me.

She said to me: 'I gave up breastfeeding three months ago but I feel so guilty that I keep coming to the meetings.'

Such is the power of guilt!

Preparation for bottle-feeding

The formula used in bottle-feeding is made either from cow's milk, goat's milk or soya beans. The ingredients in the formula are altered in an attempt to make it more like breastmilk.

There are a variety of bottles and teats to choose from. The most important thing to check is the rate of flow of the milk. It should come out as a steady drip. If it comes in a stream, your baby may get too much too quickly and spit it out. If it is too slow, she may tire before she gets enough milk.

Sterilisation – a must

It is essential that you use some form of sterilising process for all bottle-feeding equipment, to reduce the risk of illness. The most commonly used processes involve boiling water or chemicals.

To sterilise by boiling, place your equipment in a large saucepan, cover it with water and bring to the boil. Leave the equipment in the boiling water for at least five minutes. Allow the water to cool, then remove the parts and leave them to drain.

Anti-bacterial chemicals come in liquid or tablet form. Place the feeding equipment in a container, and cover it with the prepared chemical solution (ensure you follow the manufacturer's directions closely). Put the lid on the container and leave it for the recommended time, then remove your equipment.

Steam and microwave sterilisers are also available.

Making up the formula

1 Boil water in your electric jug and allow it to cool before mixing the formula.
2 Follow the manufacturer's instructions exactly when adding the formula.
3 Stand the bottle in warm water or in a bottle warmer with a thermostat control.
4 Check the temperature of the feed by shaking some onto your wrist. It should be just warm.

How to bottle-feed

To commence a feed, place the teat against your baby's lips. As she starts to suck, angle the bottle upwards to keep the neck full and prevent her sucking in air. If she stops sucking, sit her up and gently rub her back to bring up any wind.

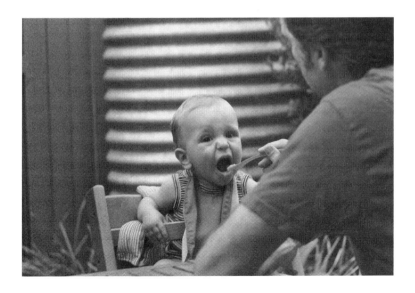

Safety facts

- Don't heat the bottle in the microwave. This could result in uneven heating and possible injury.
- Prepared bottles should be stored in the refrigerator for no longer than 24 hours.
- Discard any formula left in the bottle after a feed is complete.
- Check with your doctor or Child and Family Health Nurse if you are concerned that your baby is not getting enough milk or if you have problems with any aspect of bottle-feeding.

Now that your baby is feeding, let's consider a routine job resulting from a side effect of feeding.

A change of nappy

You will probably be amazed by how often your baby needs a change. It seems like a full-time job keeping them dry and comfortable. In the first few months babies may need changing at least eight times a day. As Tom said, it's another task that builds a connection between parent and child. Together with all the other repetitive duties you have as a parent, it is an important foundation for developing a relationship with your baby.

Tom's hints for dads on changing nappies

'Learn how to change my nappy. It's not rocket science, and after your first hundred you'll be an expert.

Again, see it as a time for you and me to connect – don't let Mum have all the fun! Sometimes it seems that mums are better at changing nappies, but this is only the result of practice.

A change table is a good investment. Make sure it satisfies the required safety standards, and never leave me unattended.'

A warm bath

Now to a parenting task most parents imagine will be pure enjoyment – bathtime.

Babies don't need a daily bath. As long as their extremities are washed with warm water, they only need to be bathed a couple of times a week. Having a bath with you or your partner can be fun and once again a great way to connect with your baby.

Julie's hints for dads on bathtime

'Learn how to bath me. Most hospitals have a training session for new parents before they leave. Make a point of being there.

Try having a bath with me – you'll love it! Make sure Mum is there to take over the drying – it's too dangerous to try the whole thing on your own. If you haven't got a bath, try showering with me. Make sure you have a non-slip mat on the floor. If you use a baby bath, never leave me unattended. And it's a good idea to have everything you need within reach.

Be prepared – I'll kick you out of the bath as soon I grow and need room for my toys.'

There is no doubt that parenting in the early days involves a number of simple, repetitive tasks that are essential. Each day is a repeat of the day before – feeding, changing, holding, rocking, bathing, changing, holding, rocking, etc., etc., etc.

Not only are these tasks essential for your baby's survival and development, they are critical in establishing the foundation for a strong relationship. It is important to see them as opportunities for connection. Yes, at times they can be tedious – even boring! At times you may feel that every day is just the same as the one before it. The outcomes, however, will make it all worthwhile – a healthy, happy child, and strong relationships with both your baby and your partner.

Sleep

If new parents could be granted one wish, it would be that their baby is healthy. If they had a second wish, it would probably be that she would sleep all through the night, from the first day she comes home! Unfortunately, this wish rarely comes true.

If you ever want evidence that babies are individuals, look at their sleep patterns. It is known that, on average, babies sleep about 16 hours in a 24-hour period. This could mean that your baby will sleep anywhere from 9 to 20 hours a day. Frustratingly, your baby may sleep for 20 hours in the first few days and then switch to the other end of the spectrum. If your baby seems healthy and is thriving, then she is getting enough sleep.

Most babies are awake for some period during the night. This is certainly a test for new parents. It is recommended that you accept your baby's routine and share the discomfort of broken sleep – realising it will end. You may hear or read about an approach called 'controlled crying'. This technique involves allowing your baby to cry for a period, checking on their safety, allowing the crying to continue for a longer period, and checking on them again. The theory is that the baby will develop some capacity to settle themselves. This approach has the potential to increase the stress on both baby and parents, and is definitely *not* recommended for babies under six months. Its usefulness for older babies is also increasingly questioned.

Remember, teenagers don't want to sleep with their parents and are well known for their ability to sleep for extremely long periods.

Sleeping safely

There are a number of recommendations to reduce the chance of cot death or Sudden Infant Death Syndrome (SIDS). They include:

1   Sleep your baby on the back from birth, not on her tummy or side.

2   Sleep your baby with her face uncovered (do not use doonas, pillows, lambs wool, bumpers or soft toys).

3   Avoid exposing your baby to tobacco smoke before birth and after.

4   Provide a safe sleeping environment (safe cot, safe mattress, safe bedding).

5   Sleep your baby in her own safe sleeping environment next to your bed for the first six to twelve months of life.

When you watch your baby sleep in those early months, you may be amazed at how restless she appears. It can seem that she is continually twitching and about to wake up. Babies' sleep patterns are different from adult patterns in the first few months – in particular, there is little difference in brain activity between a baby's sleeping and waking periods. Your baby will gradually fall into periods of deep sleep, but her patterns will only start to resemble those of an adult by the end of the first year.

Brendon's tips for dads on sleep

'Be prepared! I don't really understand your need for sleep – to be honest I don't really care. And I don't know the difference between night and day.

If possible, take a couple of weeks off work when I arrive home. Learn and practise settling techniques. These include wrapping, rocking, patting, soft music and, of course, the old favourite, walking the floor and singing or humming to me.

Share the waking times with Mum. It will be easier if you work as a team – and it will give us more time together. Remember that you and Mum may get angry with me. This is normal if your sleep is continually disrupted. Talking about how you feel will help.

Grab every bit of support and help you can get. If nothing else, it will reassure you that I'm okay.'

Growth and development just right for them

You are now aware that babies vary in their need for sleep. A similar variation applies to their general growth and development.

'Sitting in this room with my six-month-old peers, one thing is obvious – we are all different. We're different in size; different in looks; different in what we can and can't do. Stephanie can sit on her own. Brendon is rolling around. Julie is doing amazing things with her feet – she's trying to get them into her mouth. Me, I can only just grab my foot; I can't roll very well and I've no chance of sitting on my own.'
Tom, 6 months

Your baby is unique. She will grow and develop at her own rate. The variation in growth and development may be general, or it might only be noticeable in one specific area.

Babies are born with many skills. They are able to see and hear, and they can communicate. The greatest skill they have is an amazing ability to learn.

There is a pattern to their development: they move from simple to more complex behaviours. Their achievements are referred to as 'milestones'. Milestones are what you may expect your baby to be doing within a certain age range. For example, your baby will follow a rattle with her eyes any time between one and three months. Premature babies are generally behind in most areas of development, but most catch up by school age – if not sooner.

There are many books and websites that provide more detailed information on developmental milestones. You can also ask medical and nursing staff for some information on milestones when you visit them for 'checkups'.

It is normal for parents to compare their baby with her peers. This can cause anxiety – which is often increased by the tiresome comparisons made by relatives and friends. Unless grandparents have kept a daily record in writing or on video, their memory should generally not be trusted.

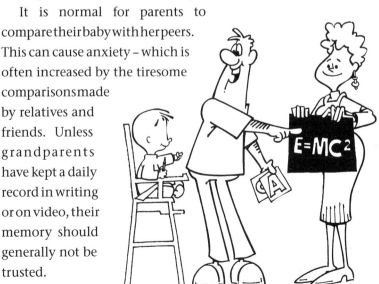

Watching your baby grow and develop is a magical experience. To be part of that experience is a privilege, but it does bring responsibilities. The responsibilities don't relate to buying the latest and best toys; rather, they involve your role in daily care, stimulating interaction and, of course, love.

What babies like

'My first memories were of faces. At first they were blurry, but after a while they became Mum and Dad. I soon saw that there was all this colour in my room – mobiles, wallpaper and toys tied to my cot. This was great, but it was Mum's and Dad's faces that fascinated me. Dad would smile a lot as he changed me. He could also change the shape of his face as he sang to me. As I grew, I made faces back at him. He would be delighted and call Mum to show her what I could do. You should have seen his reaction when I first imitated his smile!'
Joel, 6 months

'I remember Dad and Mum taking me to the toyshop when I was about six weeks old. Dad wanted to buy me this huge train set. Mum convinced Dad to wait a while and they settled on this board thing that made all kinds of noises. It was interesting. The sounds I remember most, though, were made by Dad and Mum. Dad would tell me all sorts of stories. He'd talk about work and let me know all the football results. I didn't care what he talked about, I just loved the sound of his voice.

I also remember that both Mum and Dad sang to me. I kept practising and eventually I learnt to make sounds other than "waaah". Hey, one day we may be a famous trio – or I may become a sports commentator.'
Jessica, 6 months

'I loved being held. Dad and Mum were hesitant at first – holding me as if I would easily break. After we got used to each other, cuddling became regular and enjoyable – at feed times, change times, bath times and, I have to admit, crying times. I can remember Dad walking up and down in the middle of the night with me in his arms. I know he was tired and he did mumble a lot, but he held me as if I was even more important than sleep.

Mum and Dad both went to a massage class and I was the lucky beneficiary. The way they stroked my hands and feet in those early days was pure enjoyment. As I got older, they tried a body massage after my bath. Hey, that was heaven. It not only made me feel good, it taught me about my body. It also taught me about Mum and Dad – they are so special.'

Tom, 6 months

Your face, voice and touch are the best 'toys' your baby can experience. In your daily interaction, you and your partner can provide all the stimulation your baby needs in those early days. Toys are fine, but they are 'extras'.

We have all heard that children learn from their parents. This is true – from birth on. They may not be able to copy everything, but your involvement and interaction is helping them learn.

Touch is a type of interaction that is sometimes undervalued. Babies vary in how much physical contact they enjoy. Some can't get enough, while others seem to get restless if held or nursed for too long. Regardless, touch is important for their development.

Brain development

Research consistently reinforces the importance of a child's early experiences for their brain development. This is well summarised by Sean Brotherson:

'Perhaps no aspect of child development is so miraculous and transformative as the development of a child's brain. Brain development allows a child to develop the abilities to crawl, speak, eat, laugh and walk. Healthy development of a child's brain is built on the small moments that parents and caregivers experience as they interact with a child.'

He also identifies some important myths and facts regarding brain development:

'Brain Development – Myth or Fact?

Myth At birth the brain is fully developed, just like one's heart or stomach.

Fact Most of the brain's cells are formed before birth, but most of the connections among cells are made during infancy and early childhood.

Myth The brain's development depends entirely on the genes with which you are born.

Fact Early experience and interaction with the environment are most critical in a child's brain development.

Myth A toddler's brain is less active than the brain of a college student.

Fact A 3-year-old's brain is twice as active as an adult's brain.

Myth Talking to a baby is not important because he or she can't understand what you are saying.

Fact Talking to young children establishes foundations for learning language during early critical periods when learning is easiest for a child.

Myth Children need special help and specific educational toys to develop their brainpower.

Fact What children need most is loving care and new experiences, not special attention or costly toys. Talking, singing, playing and reading are some of the key activities that build a child's brain.

Now let's hear from another 'expert' – Jessica:

'Dad's been reading me stuff about my brain and how it develops. Of course, he thinks I'm going to be a genius. He told me that I was born with an "immature brain" – yeah, right! Apparently I had most of my brain cells but what was missing was the connections between the cells. It seems that now these connections are critical. Dad says I was "born to learn", and that stuff he and Mum do will make all the difference.

When he changes my nappy, baths me, holds me and talks to me, he is actually helping my brain develop. And I thought he was just having a good time! Even when he sings to me, he is apparently helping my language skills develop. He then got heavy and said that my brain development is affected by my experiences of love, security, trust and stimulation. I guess he was trying to say that what he does and how he does it will help my brain. So far I have no complaints.'

Jessica, 6 months

As Jessica so beautifully put it, your baby's experiences in her early years will affect the development of her brain. In the first three years, most of the core brain structure will develop. Your baby is an active 'player' in her brain's development: she is biologically prepared to learn, and her interactions with you contribute greatly to her development.

Parents also play an important part by responding to their baby and, importantly, meeting their child's basic needs during daily care. The routine of holding, feeding, changing nappies, talking, touching, smiling, singing, bathing and walking the floor is the most critical ingredient for the development of your baby's brain. Mobiles, visits to the park and toys are an added bonus.

The early days are critical for the development of your baby's brain, and the wonderful thing is that good quality care and love provide the best start.

The key message is: *you are important, and your involvement from the beginning can make a difference.*

Joel's tips for dads on growth and development

'I'm an individual. I will grow and develop at my own pace, so look for my strengths – not my weaknesses.

Don't underestimate the importance of daily caring in my development. This helps build my skills and a connection with you. Toys are good, but I prefer your smile, touch and voice.

Don't wait until I can kick a football; play with me now – gently but often.

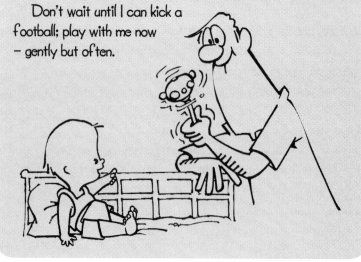

If you think I'm falling behind in my development, get some advice. If something is wrong, early intervention produces the best results. You are important to me. What you do now will make a difference.'

To feel safe

Protecting your baby is an instinct you share with all new parents. Keeping her safe is a priority, and there are some practical things you can do right from the start.

Keep your home free from ongoing conflict and violence

As we have already stressed many times, your relationship with your partner is important to your child – and to her development. Relationships with high levels of conflict, particularly conflict accompanied by violence, can have serious long-term consequences for your child.

Violence between couples is all too frequently accompanied by violence towards children – which is also a significant risk factor impacting on all stages of their development.

With all the changes and challenges you face on the journey to becoming parents, there is the chance that conflict may begin or increase. It is important to recognise and address this issue right from the beginning.

The Queensland Centre for Domestic and Family Violence Research state in their Factsheet Series:

★ 'Thinking that babies and toddlers are too young to be affected by domestic and family violence is a mistake.'

★ 'Living with ongoing domestic or family violence affects the development of babies' and toddlers' brains. These effects can be permanent.'

★ 'Babies as young as six weeks show clear disturbance in response to domestic and family violence.'

★ 'Babies react strongly to tension, fear and aggression in their environment.'

Conflict will occur in all relationships – how you deal with it is the critical factor. We have already recommended that you deal with any conflict as soon as it occurs – don't let it fester. Unresolved conflict will damage relationships. At this time of stress, it is critical that you have a method of swiftly addressing any issues with your partner, so they don't escalate to a point where they affect your relationship. If you act quickly and positively, you will reap the benefits for years to come. Some useful strategies are:

★ If you have a disagreement with your partner, talk about it when you are both calm – not in the heat of an argument.

★ Address the issue – without attacking your partner.

★ Listen to how your partner feels.

★ Be willing to change what you can about your behaviour.

★ Remember what you love and respect about your partner and acknowledge it to them.

If ongoing conflict or violence are issues in your relationship, acknowledge this, seek professional help and *remove them from your life.*

Buy safe equipment for your baby

When purchasing anything for your baby, make sure you ask yourself 'Is it safe?' You will need somewhere for your baby to sleep, a means of transporting her, and probably a change table. Cots, strollers and car restraints must conform to a set of standards. Detailed information regarding standards for baby equipment is readily available from Kidsafe, Choice and state government Fair Trading offices (see 'Resources' at the back of this book).

If you buy new equipment, it should come with a clear statement that it conforms to the appropriate safety standards. If you are buying or are given second-hand equipment, check that it meets the standards by contacting one of the above organisations, or ask your midwife or doctor for information.

Train your pets

If you have pets, it is important to plan for the arrival of the baby. Make sure you consider hygiene and possible negative reactions to the 'intruder'. Preparing a dog which lives inside for a move outside is a recommended strategy, and this is best achieved before your baby comes home. Cats love warm places, so be aware that they may try to curl up with your baby in the cot or bassinet. Show your animals that they are important, despite the changes in their routines. Provide affection and some special time so they remain a part of your family.

Be alert to risks

Unfortunately, accidents do occur – even with a newborn baby – so it is worthwhile doing a safety check on your house. Smoke detectors are an essential investment, and a strategically placed night light can make responding to your baby during the dark hours a safer experience. Examine each room and consider possible risks. As with many areas of parenting, planning and preparation can make a big difference.

As your baby grows, the potential risks increase. One minute she is lying quietly on the change table; the next she has discovered rolling.

Tony: I remember when my first baby was about four months old. I was changing her nappy and turned to get something. In an instant she rolled off the change table and landed heavily on the floor. She was motionless for what seemed like ages, and initially I froze. I picked her up and called my partner. By then she was screaming and we took her to the hospital. Thank God she was okay. I felt awful, but I learnt a valuable lesson on being prepared for the unexpected results of growth.

Babies are at their most vulnerable in the early months, and this is when you need to be aware of possible dangers and remain vigilant. As children grow, they will have accidents – hopefully minor. As parents, we need to try and minimise the risks by 'childproofing' the house, while also recognising that it is important for children to explore and to challenge their environment.

Have your child immunised against diseases

Immunisation is an important safety issue for your baby. The effectiveness of immunisation in protecting children from life-threatening diseases is now generally acknowledged and widely accepted. However, some parents are still concerned about the possible side effects of immunisation. If you have questions or concerns, talk to your doctor.

Group reflections on the first six months

'Both Mum and Dad knew very little about me when I was born. They worked together and soon it didn't matter who changed me, settled me or played with me. It was great having two people who knew how to care for me. I know it made a difference.'

'My dad always made me feel special. Even when he went back to work, he still made time for me. I looked forward to him coming home, and so did Mum. I wasn't an easy baby but Dad and Mum seemed to cope. Dad often did the morning shift with me. He would get me up and look after me so that Mum could stay in bed a little longer. They were great times.'

'I'm a twin – the more important one of course. Mum and Dad were in a state of shock for the first few months. Working as a team was a matter of survival for all of us. I know I'm going to love being a twin. I'll have someone to blame for any mistakes!'

'The one thing I want to say about parenting is – it's about me, me, me. Dad and Mum have treated me as the centre of their universe. I feel special and I appreciate what they have done for me.'

'I recommend that all parents get together a collection of decent DVDs for those long and lonely nights.'

Summary

★ Babies need you to respond to their crying as well as look after the basic things like food, baths, nappy changes and sleep.

★ They also need to develop at their own pace and, very importantly, be kept safe.

★ Caring regularly for your baby in all these ways makes them feel loved and secure and supports their development. It also helps you connect with your child.

★ The challenges for you during this part of the journey are real (and sometimes tedious). The rewards for your involvement will last a lifetime.

★ Keep reminding yourself how important your relationship with your partner is for your child's development – practise your communication skills and address any conflict positively as soon as it occurs.

8 Connecting with your baby

'This is it: the ultimate in being a father – the lasting deep relationship you develop with your child. It is a feeling that is hard to describe – it's all about being connected, the love you share, the enjoyment, the recognition, the care you give. It is a lifetime investment, a connection that travels with you everywhere you go. You never lose it. I remember going to a fathering group just after Jacob was born and the facilitator (who was a grandfather) was asked by one of the participants what to him was the most important thing to focus on as a father. He replied that it was staying connected and keeping the relationship alive through the good and bad times and the challenges and difficulties – to keep the focus on the relationship.'

Brad, 29

In this chapter, we explore a range of issues regarding your relationship with your child. Although we have covered this from some perspectives, we will now look in more depth at the importance of connecting with your baby and how you can build this connection from the time he is born.

We will start by hearing reflections on being a father from a group of men who have older children. They were asked to discuss their experiences of being a dad and, for some, a grandparent as well.

What older dads say

'My children are grown up and have moved out of home. I think back to my early days as a dad and realise that I missed out on a lot. I am a truck driver and right from the beginning I was away from home for a lot of their young lives. Mary was great with the kids and I thought I would be needed as they got older for discipline and sports stuff. I didn't think I needed to be involved much when they were babies. What happened was that I never really got close to them. Sure I provided some back-up to Mary when I was home, but I was just the loud voice when it was needed, supporting her in what she did. I didn't realise what I missed out on until my eldest girl had a baby. I got the chance to care for him and loved every minute of it. Mary and my daughter were surprised at how much I enjoyed it. I'm closer to my grandson than I ever was with my children.'

Frank, 56

'I know what you mean. I didn't get involved much until they could kick a football or needed help with their homework. I saw how close Janette was to the children and how they would talk to her about anything. Me, I was the last resort if they wanted a different answer. I never got that closeness and it was what I wanted with my children as they grew up. If I had my time over again I would do things differently. I think the closeness Janette had with them came from what she did. She did all the basic stuff when they were little and that seemed to make the difference. I hope I get the same chance you've had with your grandchild – a second chance.'

Ben, 51

'For me, it was different. I worked shift work and Helen went back to work three months after our first was born. I had to do the basic stuff. At first it was hard but I got to love the time with my kids, particularly when they were little. Even when their mum was home, they would still come to me if they got hurt or wanted a cuddle. Of course they did that to Helen as well, but for some reason I was usually the first choice. I think it was because I did everything with them that needed to be done when they were babies and I'm sure that was why we were so close. I'm still close to them and can't wait to have a grandchild. There is something special about holding and caring for a little one.'

Tom, 53

'Growing up I hardly knew my father. It wasn't until I left home and started to meet him for a game of golf and a beer that I realised what a great bloke he was! He was easy to talk to and I really looked forward to seeing him. I convinced myself that things would be different with my children. I wanted to know them and for them to know me before they left home, but it didn't turn out that way. I started a business just before my first child was born and it took me away from home in their early years. By the stage I had more time for my family, it was too late. I didn't know how to interact with them and they had other interests. I now realise that having a successful business did not give me what I really wanted – a good relationship with my children. I think my lack of involvement also affected my relationship with their mum. I left it all to her and it wore thin after a while, but I couldn't get off the roller-coaster of work. I realised what was important after the damage was done.'

Ray, 59

Many fathers of grown up children regret that they missed an opportunity to make that early connection with their baby, a connection that provides both the foundation and the pathway for a lifetime relationship. The causes of this lack of connection are many and varied – social expectations of the father's role as provider first; lack of understanding of the importance of their early involvement; the common view that mothers are more important to babies; and work pressures (not being available at critical times).

The dads who did connect report a different picture of ongoing closeness with their children and commonly a stronger relationship with their partner.

So what makes the difference?

Understanding the importance of this connection

The first step in connecting is to believe it is important. We hear and read a lot about a mother 'bonding' with her baby, now more commonly referred to as 'attachment'. Books, research and services have for many years been devoted to the relationship between mother and baby. They have emphasised its importance, studied the implications of good and poor attachment, and at times have created a romantic image of the process.

What happens between a mother and her baby is often described like something in a Mills and Boon novel. This 'something' happens when a woman gives birth – just as 'something' happens when two strangers in a novel look across the dance floor and ZAP, they are instantly in love. Too often the adult scenario is based on physical attraction, even lust. For the poor mum waiting for the ZAP to produce some kind of instant bond with her baby, this could be a non-event. We can carry this further and imagine a nurse patrolling the maternity unit, eyeing off all the new mums and saying 'You have bonded, you haven't'.

As mothers will tell you, the connection with their baby can be very different. Like any other relationship, the genuine bond, or attachment, comes in time and is the result of the touching, walking the floor, feeding, changing, and the giving of time and self to the other party – in this case, the baby. In the case of fathers, the importance of connecting has been studied only recently, and rarely. Its importance is often relegated to 'Oh yes, and fathers can bond too' or 'Babies can be attached to their fathers as well' as a footnote to a chapter, or at the back of a book on parenting.

Is it any wonder that some dads struggle with the importance of connecting with their baby? The message, too often, is still 'forget the baby stage, you become visible and important when it all gets too much for Mum, or the children need someone to play with them, chastise them or take them to sport'.

The bonding that results from the basic care of a baby is recognised by anyone who has studied or supported mothers in those early days as a parent. It is recognised that the mother's life experiences, current circumstances and the temperament of the baby impact on the mother–child relationship. What is not questioned is the importance of the relationship.

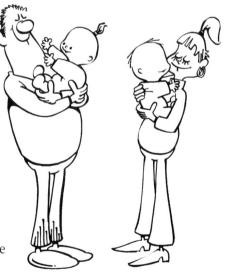

But what about the father–child relationship?

FASCINATING FACTS ABOUT FATHERS

- Fathers who take on more responsibility for the daily care of their infants have been found to show more responsiveness to them.

- Mothers and fathers are equally anxious about leaving their babies in someone else's care.

- Mothers and fathers both adjust their speech patterns when talking to babies. Both speak more slowly, use shorter phrases, imitate and repeat themselves more often than when talking to adults.

- Fathers who sing to their children have been found to increase their pitch and frequency range even more than mothers do.

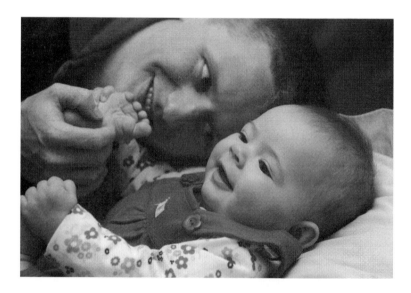

If you are to connect with your baby, a good start is believing that it is important. Research and our experience indicate that it is, and that connecting can make a real difference to your child. According to Michael Lamb, Professor of Psychology at Cambridge University, and Charlie Lewis, Professor of Psychology at the University of Lancaster in the UK, 'The establishment of attachment relationships between children and parents constitutes one of the most important aspects of human social and emotional development.'

Both mothers and fathers are important contributors to this process. When fathers are in tune with their babies' signals (e.g. crying, smiling), and respond sensitively and appropriately (e.g. soothing by rocking, smiling back and talking to baby), their babies will see them as predictable and reliable, and they will develop secure relationships with their dads. It is this early stage of responding sensitively to your baby that provides the foundation for your long-lasting relationship.

Michael Lamb and Charlie Lewis point out that there are four developmental phases in the establishment of attachment relationships. Two of these are relevant here:

Months 1 and 2: Indiscriminate social responsiveness, where the baby is not able to differentiate between the people who form part of his social world.

Months 3 to 7: Discriminating sociability, where the infant is able to recognise the differences between people in his social world. He can now recognise the different patterns and expressions he experiences with his mother and father, so it is at this age that you start to make a difference to your baby. He begins to get to know you by the way you interact, respond, touch, play, etc. Although it might not appear so at the time, the nature of your interactions now will make a difference to your relationship in the future.

FASCINATING FACTS ABOUT FATHERS

- Fathers can be just as sensitive and responsive to their young children as mothers can. Providing sensitive and responsive care – care that takes account of the needs of the child and of the child's own patterns and daily rhythms (e.g. their need for sleep or attention) – leads to positive outcomes for infants.

- Babies become attached to both fathers and mothers, it depends on responding lovingly and sensitively and providing enjoyable and playful stimulation. Research shows that security of attachment is a strong predictor of positive outcomes for children.

- Engagement in play by fathers, and especially their play sensitivity (having a warm interactional style, engaging in reciprocal interactions, and providing age-appropriate stimulation), are significant predictors of the nature of a child's peer relationships later in life.

- '… 10 of the 14 (longitudinal) studies controlling for maternal involvement and employing different source data (i.e. the information about father involvement was provided by someone other than the father) found positive correlates of paternal involvement' with longer-term outcomes for children (e.g. positive school attitudes).

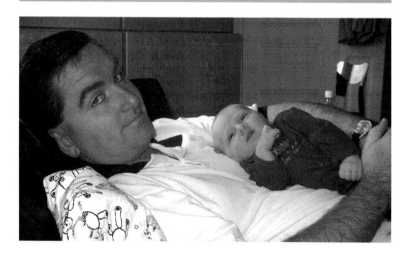

What can you do?

The answer to this is simple – be involved. How you achieve this will vary, but here are some hints:

- Believe that you are important to your baby.
- Understand that what you do as a dad will impact on outcomes for your baby. Perhaps this might mean reframing the way you think about your time with your baby – all interaction is an opportunity for connection.
- Consult one of the many books on fathers (see Resources at the end of the book) for up-to-date findings on the impact fathers have on their children.
- Talk to other fathers about what they see as important in this role.

What to do to connect with your baby

As we said in the chapter on Pregnancy, you can start to connect even before your baby is born. You can start to think about your baby, feel him move, talk to him and even see him on the ultrasound. You can attend appointments with health professionals, go to antenatal classes and take an active role during the period of the pregnancy. The connection has begun.

You will probably be present at the birth and experience a range of emotions as your partner gives birth. You will see and possibly hold your baby following the birth, and experience an overwhelming feeling of love. This strengthens your connection.

You have only just begun. What you do when your baby comes home will impact on the start you have made in connecting with your baby. There is no difference between you and your partner in what is important and what will impact on your connection or attachment to your baby. As pointed out in Chapter 7, the importance of providing the basic care your baby needs to developing a relationship with your baby applies equally to both you and your partner.

So you need to get involved, to get your hands dirty from the beginning. It is the touching, the holding, the walking the floor and the responding to your baby that makes the connection. It is also the social interaction that you engage in while doing these tasks. For example, when picking your baby up from his pram, there is the opportunity to engage in conversation or to mimic your baby's sounds. Start to play with your baby – put him on a rug on the floor, lie down with him, and so on.

A baby is a lot more competent than you might think. Babies are not blobs! Their sensory systems are extremely well developed at birth, and a baby thrives on stimulation. A newborn has:

* a highly developed sense of touch – he is capable of removing an irritant from his skin using either a hand or a foot

* discrimination in taste and smell – just like adults, they prefer sweet-tasting things

* discrimination between different types of sounds and where they come from

* considerable visual discrimination – babies can turn and focus on different light sources, track moving objects and perceive distance and depth.

But a baby's capacities are much more highly developed and complex than just straightforward sensory discrimination. Newborns are able to imitate adults who poke out their tongues or blink at them, and are actually able to turn their heads in

response to different types of stimuli. This capacity to imitate you lasts for life – look for it emerging in complete form when your child gives a speech about you at your 50th birthday!

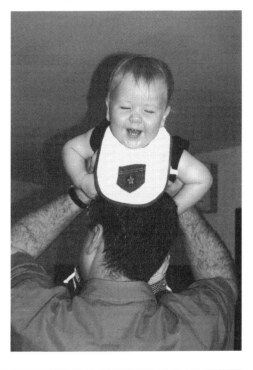

From around three months, infants are able to coordinate eyes and hands, and can reach out to touch or hold something of interest – or, more commonly, put things into their mouths.

'I was amazed at what Julian seemed capable of. I used to watch him while he was asleep, and the best time of all was when he was waking up. I have some fantastic videos of his little antics while he was coming back into my world. Well, noticing I was there. I had never thought about what babies might be capable of – I had it in mind that my relationship would have to wait until Julian was walking. Not so! I keep telling other dads-to-be to get set

> for full action from the beginning. I was convinced he was advanced when he began smiling at me at about four weeks. No-one believed me, but he just kept doing it. I still feel a sense of happiness when I think that I shared his first smile with him.'
>
> David, 31

Babies begin to smile enthusiastically at parents and others at about four to six weeks. When this happens, you can certainly get more satisfaction and enjoyment from play. What father doesn't experience pleasure from their baby smiling at them? At about four to six months, babies are able to recognise their parents consistently and respond to them in characteristic ways (you will know what these are). There is dispute about this, with some saying that it actually occurs much earlier. You might also note some hint of a negative reaction to strangers at around six months.

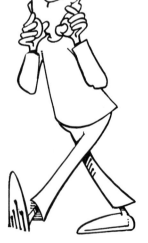

Your baby will also be sensitive to your voice and the individual ways in which you respond to him – how long you let him cry, how you hold him, what you do before and after feeds and before and after his sleep, and the characteristic way in which you change his nappy (a good time to have a chat and ask your baby a question or two!).

There is no reason why you can't begin to interact socially with your baby and find ways to stimulate him from the first few days onwards. Playing games, talking and describing things, amusing him with bright, moving and perhaps audible objects, poking funny faces, hugging him, being physical, getting on the floor and rolling around, tickling, encouraging him to follow or track visual and auditory objects and to reach out and explore things – these are all things you can do. Plenty of face-to-face contact, talking, smiling, singing and hand clapping are other things that infants enjoy.

As your baby gets older, you can find ways to allow him freedom to explore, and to allow you some freedom to do things while retaining auditory and physical contact. A rug on the floor, a bouncinette and an infant seat (when his neck is strong enough) can all help. You can attach a mobile to the back of a bouncinette, so that every time your baby bounces, the mobile moves. These little tricks can be useful before feeds and during nappy changes and baths, but can be counterproductive if engaged in too vigorously after feeds or just before bedtime.

What can you do?

- Be creative in how you interact with your baby – look for ways to stimulate and be responsive to him. One father used to sing to his baby when he first came home in the afternoon. It fulfilled two purposes. First, it was stimulating for his baby, providing a pathway for connecting and developing their relationship; and second, he found it helped him switch off from work and increased his energy levels.
- Do the basic chores of caring and responding to your baby. Yes, responding to your baby while doing these 'tasks' is a key part of being a parent.

- Be an active member of the 'parenting team' – not a support person to your partner. When you are having a good connection in terms of stimulating and playing with your baby, this can be used to change the mood of your baby and of your household. It also serves to increase the energy level in your relationship with your partner – something that is vital to a team approach.
- Develop a routine in the way you and your partner care for your baby; ensure there are opportunities for both of you to get involved in the different aspects of your baby's day-to-day life.

Being involved with your child from the start, and maintaining this involvement, are fundamental to connecting with your child and having a rewarding long-term relationship with him. Your relationship with your partner is another important indicator of how well you will maintain the connection with your child. If you adopt a teamwork approach, there is more chance you will continue to be involved.

Nevertheless, there is no doubt that the very real pressures of life will challenge the level of your early and ongoing involvement with your child. The impact of work, and ways of dealing with the competing demands of family and work, are discussed in the next chapter.

Summary

★ We have covered two major issues in this chapter: why it is important for you to be connected with your child, and how you can establish and maintain this connection.

★ It is critical that you recognise that you are as important to your child's development as your partner.

★ Remember that babies are much more capable than many of us expect.

★ Connecting with your child begins during pregnancy and continues with the daily care you give your infant when he is very young.

★ As he gets a bit older, he will respond to your stimulation and play, including talking, smiling, cuddling, singing and rolling around on the floor.

9 Integrating work and fatherhood

The fathers we've had conversations with have expressed mixed views about whether it is more or less difficult for fathers today to balance their work and family lives than it was in the past. New fathers commonly say they want to be involved with their children and, for some, this means they want to be more involved than their own fathers were.

Involvement can mean different things to different fathers. For some it will mean making sure they spend time with their baby; for others it will mean getting involved in the day-to-day care, changing nappies and so on; for yet others it will mean being available at times that they see as being more critical (e.g. late afternoon), to connect and listen to their child, or simply to be there with them. And for others it might mean making considerable adjustments to their work by adapting their career aspirations and work responsibilities, or reducing their hours (e.g. by working part-time, or taking paternity or parental leave), so that they can take responsibility for the care of their baby for a significant part of the week. As we highlighted earlier, more families are now choosing the option of having both parents work part-time, so they can share the care of their child.

Fathers commonly experience some pressure – either in terms of meeting their own expectations or in meeting the expectations of others. Few men report that their workplaces are highly responsive to the needs of fathers. Graeme's research in Australian organisations has shown that nearly 45 per cent of fathers feel that if they access flexible work practices to engage more actively as a father, it will be interpreted as a lack of commitment to their job. The challenge of balancing work and family is something that many fathers figure out for themselves, with little support from their workplace or from other fathers. They don't have a boss telling them it is important that they take time off when they have a new baby, that it is important to be available and accessible to their child, and nor are new fathers encouraged to reflect on what their priorities are or could be in the future. The possibility that workplaces could operate in this way is not such an unusual idea. Short-term paternity leave (e.g. for two weeks) is now commonly accepted in many countries, and fathers are fully expected to take this leave.

For many fathers, too, the challenge of establishing new work and family priorities becomes an internal struggle – mixed with anxiety, a sense of pressure, and at times guilt. In our experience, guilt does not work well for fathers. A much better motivator is to focus on what is in it for fathers – what are the opportunities for them if they are actively involved with their children? And, the latest research shows that this can be good for workplaces as well!

In this chapter we focus on three of the common work and family challenges experienced by fathers:

1 finding time for family, work and themselves

2 switching off from work and being available, or 'present', when they are at home

3 making work work for them – finding creative ways to make changes at work that will help them be the kind of fathers they would like to be.

Finding time for family, work and you

Recognising the competing demands of your work, family and personal lives is an essential beginning. Too often work demands just 'happen' and the impact is upon you before you realise it. Being aware of the competing demands and discussing these with your partner can lead to creative solutions and positive outcomes.

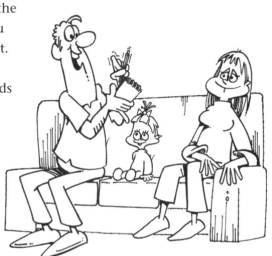

What dads say about time

'Jodie keeps telling me that I need to reduce my hours and that I need to spend more time with the children. This is not about who does what – she is not hounding me about doing more housework or taking more responsibility for James – it is simply about my being there, to be with James, share time with him and enjoy being a father. This is still very difficult for me because of my work demands. There is a big change project going on at work, so I am there from about 7.30 a.m. to 6.30 p.m. I have to be there to get the work done. And then I have to work at nights as well as I have too many interruptions during the day to get through all my emails. Great this virtual office thing – you can be available 24/7 no matter where you are! Our organisation expects you to answer emails overnight and then there is the BUS that hits you every now and then. The BUS is the Bloody US – our company is based in the United States and my boss over there expects me to be available on his time zone as well.'

Brad, 36

'Yes, time and what priority I am giving to each aspect of my life are critical issues for me. How this hit me was that I suddenly realised I didn't have much time for myself after we had Luke. I had a lot of activities in my life as well as a very demanding job. What helped me was that I did a small audit on how I was spending my time – as a way of checking on how my life was being played out. This helped sort out my priorities. I also realised that if I was going to be an effective father who was around for the long term, I needed to look after myself as well.'

Andrew, 31

'I would like to be there more for Harry. Louise and I have had many discussions about this. I suppose it all goes down to not having total control over when we had Harry. Time was running out for us and we were still not where we wanted to be financially. With Louise not working, we now have only one income. This has meant that I have had to pick up extra work in overtime at the factory as a way to make ends meet. This means I have less time at home

189

during the week than I would like. I try to make up for it on weekends, and I do a lot of phoning home during the day to check in, to stay connected with what is happening.'

Kevin, 38

'We realised before we had Samantha that something was going to have to give when she arrived. We had seen this happen in the lives of two of our closest friends – and they warned us. So, we made a plan. This involved me adjusting my priorities and looking for ways to reduce my hours at work. I approached my boss and workgroup with a proposal, we discussed it and put it in place for a trial period. And it has worked – I now spend on average ten hours less time at work than I did before Samantha arrived. You know what? The sky hasn't fallen in and work is still getting done. I also feel much better within myself having these two major priorities in my life.'

Luke, 29

What can you do?

One option is to evaluate how you currently spend your time – to get an idea of your patterns and to see if there are opportunities for you to change them or to improve the alignment between what you would like and what is currently happening. It is also a good idea to review your time patterns on a regular basis, e.g. every couple of months.

TIMES diary

You can review how you currently spend your time by completing the TIMES diary on page 193. All you need to do is colour in each hour according to your activities over the past week (start from today and work backwards). We suggest you use blue for work time, yellow for transition time, red for individual time with your baby, green for marital or couple time, orange for time with everyone, and brown for self-time.

Note that this diary does not include everything that happens in your life – if an activity (e.g. sleep) is not covered by any of the categories, leave it out. The type of activities included here are those that have been found to make a difference to the wellbeing of fathers and to the nature of their family relationships.

W Work time (blue): This is all the time you spend on work, whether at your workplace, at home, or on the bus/train, etc.

T Transition time (yellow): This is the time when you are transitioning between home and work (e.g. in the mornings) or between work and home (e.g. in the evenings). If you are a shift worker, this transition might occur at very different times of the day. For those on regular day-time working hours, the afternoon time is sometimes called the 'arsenic hour' – late afternoon, early evening, when you have returned from work and everything is happening at home: baby is being fed and getting ready for bed, someone is looking after dinner, everyone is looking to have their needs met, etc.

I **Individual time with your baby (red):** This is the time you spend alone with your child. As we and other fathers have mentioned earlier, time alone with your child is a significant opportunity for you to establish the connection that is critical for your longer-term relationship. It is also a special time that many fathers say they value and enjoy.

M **Marital or partner time (green):** This is the time you and your partner spend together, and it is critical for developing and sustaining your relationship. Many fathers report that partner time drops off and sometimes completely disappears when they have a baby. We know from the research, though, that maintaining a high quality relationship with your partner has strong links with positive outcomes for children, and for you and your partner. We also know that this relationship can have a positive impact on your performance at work (e.g. your capacity to concentrate). What should be included here is time spent in an active way with your partner (e.g. going out to dinner, going for a walk together, having a discussion).

E **Everyone time (orange):** This is time spent together as a family when there is some focus or purpose to your activity (e.g. you could be sharing the feeding of your baby – sitting around together and being actively involved with each other). Other examples would be going for a walk together and bathing the baby together.

S **Self-time (brown):** This is the time you spend doing things for yourself. It could involve exercise or a hobby, or it could be volunteer work in the community.

Having completed the diary, spend some time reviewing it by asking yourself questions such as:

- Are there any surprises here?
- Is there more of one colour than I would have expected?
- Are there any discrepancies between what I see here and what I would like to see here (this is often called 'gap analysis')?
- What are the possibilities for changing the pattern I see?

You might also like to review the diary with your partner and ask her whether she feels there are any issues, and whether she sees any opportunities for change. You could then work together to develop a pattern that more closely fits your particular goals and needs. This could involve changing things at home (e.g. arranging for your parents to look after your child while you and your partner go out to dinner) or at work (e.g. giving more responsibility to those who report to you, to give you more flexibility to leave work early).

Time	Monday	Tuesday	Wednesday	Thursday	Friday	Saturday
AM 5–6						
6–7						
7–8						
8–9						
9–10						
10–11						
11–12						
PM 12–1						
1–2						
2–3						

3–4					
4–5					
5–6					
6–7					
7–8					
8–9					
9–10					
10–11					
11–12					
AM 12–1					
1–2					
2–3					
3–4					
4–5					

There are two other options that you could consider. First, you could reduce your overall hours by working part-time for a period of time, or taking extended parental leave (see below). The second option is to review your career aspirations. Many workplaces are exploring options for career lattices to complement the traditional career ladder. Although the majority of workplaces see career lattices as being an option that is more attractive to women, there is no reason why you couldn't explore this option in an open discussion with your immediate manager. These adjustments might also enable greater equity with your partner in combining work and family commitments (e.g. both of you might work part-time).

'I agree that organisations and the government should do more about providing options for fathers to take leave. I also think there is more that fathers could do to make this happen for them. I work for a small business and so it is highly unlikely that any of the options would ever come my way. Even so, I was able to organise to work a four-day week for a period of six months when we had our baby. It took some planning; it required this to make it happen. We began planning about eight weeks into Abbey's pregnancy. We were having dinner and fantasising what it would be like to have a child. One of my fantasies was that I would take time off work to be at home during the early months. At first both of us thought this wasn't a realistic option, but then … We looked at our finances and decided we could put away a bit more money while Abbey was still working to buffer our mortgage payments. Then we crafted a plan to put to my boss for me to work one day less each week for six months (with a 20 per cent reduction in my income). I spoke to others in the office to see how this might work without putting an extra load onto them, while still maintaining our productivity and quality of customer service. With a little bit of give and take from two other people in the office, we found a solution! When pressures did arise, there was some budget there to pay one of them to work overtime.'

Jeff, 30

'My organisation has great leave policies for mothers. I don't think they even think paternity leave is something men want, or that they would use if it was available. With the support of my manager, I decided to take them on. I wanted to take two weeks' leave when Jodie came home. This was really important to me; I have always been of the view that I should be able to take leave on full pay. My manager and I worked on the gender equity arguments and the importance of fathers, which my employer seemed to accept. The biggest stumbling block was how to back-fill my position while I was on leave for two weeks. We were able to achieve this with some flexibility in rostering over a four-week period (meaning I had to adjust some of my work hours as well) and with a small budget for employing casual staff.'

Ben, 34

It makes good sense to sort out your priorities – to ensure that the people and activities that matter to your long-term wellbeing, and to the wellbeing of your child and partner, are given priority. People who have a balanced approach to life and work are also more effective in their jobs and contribute more to their organisations.

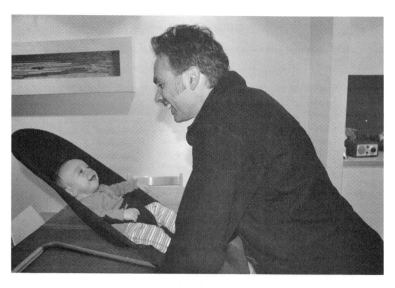

Switching off and switching in

A challenge for many men is to switch off from their jobs and be available to or present for their families – to be ready to respond, initiate interactions and so on. There are in fact three possible parts to this process. The first involves switching off from work. The second involves avoiding 'switching out' at home. If you have had a hard day at work, it might be that all you want is peace and quiet, and therefore your tendency is to disconnect from what is happening at home. The third involves 'switching in' and being actively involved in what is happening at home.

What dads say about switching off

'It is not the hours that I have a problem with. I am usually home by 5.30 in the afternoon. My problem is that I can't switch off. I still have all these work issues going around in my head. (Will we meet our targets? Why isn't that machine reliable – do we need to change our approach to maintenance?) It used to be that Maryanne and I would always have a chat when we both came home from work – we would have a cup of tea or a drink. It helped us to unwind. We used to share the little "big" things that mattered to us at work: what my boss said, what her boss didn't say, who was getting the next promotion who certainly didn't deserve it – well, really, nobody does, do they? It got a bit tedious at times, I admit, especially if either of us had major issues at work. She once said to me, "You know, Mark, our life is pretty boring at the moment. All we seem to talk about is your job and the food you like!" Now we don't even have time for these discussions. We just move straight into active mode – things have to get done

– Sam demands attention, bathing, etc. It is all go. I have to admit, I have trouble switching gears at times.'

Mark, 35

'I have some of those issues as well. However, my biggest problem is that, because my job is so physically demanding, I come home very tired and often would prefer to have dinner, watch some TV and go to bed. I can't see that I can change that – other than moving to another job. But that isn't really an option.'

Brett, 30

'Yes, I had that problem too. But Brodie and I reached a compromise. I am a morning person and so I started to look after Emily if she woke up before I went to work. I didn't admit this to Brodie at the time, but I started to get to like this pattern. Just me and Emily – talking, smiling – and I started to enjoy changing nappies. The greeting I got when she was older, when I went in to get her up, was absolutely priceless. It was an absolute joy to share her smiles and recognition first thing in the morning. I also found that this had a major impact on my mood – I was going to work on a real high! The other thing we did was that I took over more of the care on the weekends. We always have our little outings together – she really likes the hardware shop down the road! I think she might be a plumber when she grows up.'

Charlie, 25

What Charlie's comment above highlights is the value of experimenting with different family patterns. He was able to find a compromise solution that in the end turned out to be highly positive for his relationship with Brodie.

What can you do?

What you can do will depend very much on the type of job you have, how demanding it is and your level of responsibility. The suggestions below cover a range of options for fathers in different work situations.

- Set up rituals for going to work and saying good-bye. Leaving home in a good mood is critical and should set you up for a positive day at work (or, in research speak, for 'positive family to work spillover').

- Phase out of work at the end of each day. Some fathers find that starting this process about 30 minutes before they plan to leave helps them to get their work issues out of their heads.

- Don't schedule potentially tense work activities late in the day if you can avoid it.

- Develop a 'going home' ritual, which, as far as possible, includes putting a priority on leaving work at the same time each day. If you are in the car, play relaxing music or listen to a radio program that you know will help you detach from work. If you are on the bus or train, you can listen to music or read.

- Develop an 'arriving home' ritual. This might include a high energy greeting of your partner and child, with genuine focus, listening and getting a summary of the day, and then some time to yourself (e.g. to change your clothes, have a cup of tea or go for a walk in the garden). What is critical here is to give yourself time and space to wind down so that you are ready to wind up again!

- Make sure your partner's and child's needs are met when you first see them – ensure you have the focus and energy for this, and remember to use active listening.
- If you have had 'one of those days', take care of yourself and explain this to your family. Take a little time out for yourself, and then reconnect with your family.
- Put a priority on having dinner together.
- Avoid missing special family events.
- Be on call to your family at work when they need you.
- Minimise working at home. However, some fathers find that doing a little bit of work at home provides them with the flexibility to leave early every now and then.
- As far as possible, avoid making or receiving work phone calls at home, especially at critical times. Some couples find it useful to put the answering machine on when the activity level is high (e.g. when feeding, bathing or putting your baby to sleep).
- With your partner, work out a pattern of sharing the care of your child that suits your respective energy levels (e.g. you could do more on the weekends or in the mornings).
- With your partner, work out a pattern of sharing the family tasks and responsibilities – housework, paying the bills, etc. Couples find that when they have a new baby, things work better if they share the housework. Take the initiative: be pro-active in cleaning, preparing meals, and so on.
- Review all of the above suggestions and establish your own set of 'rules' (habits, values, priorities); monitor how well you stick to them.

Making work work for you!

Recent research shows that there are clear links between workplace support and the level of father involvement with their children. In a study in Sweden it was found that fathers were more likely to take parental leave if they worked in companies that had 'father-friendly' policies and practices, and workgroups that were flexible and adaptive in responding to a father's desire to take time off. It was also reported that some Swedish companies preferred to employ men who had spent time at home caring for children, on the assumption that these men would have a more diverse skill set and that they would be more likely to be able to multitask.

Findings from an Australian study show that fathers who have supervisors who are more supportive of their needs are more likely to be highly interactive with their children (e.g. playing with their children and doing day-to-day childcare tasks) and emotionally involved with their children (e.g. being affectionate, telling their children they love them).

We also know from the extensive research conducted by Professor Jeff Hill and colleagues in a global company (IBM), and replicated by Jeff and Graeme in an Australian organisation (see below), that flexible work practices enabling employees to be more actively involved in family life has benefits both for work performance and for fathers' wellbeing.

Benefits for the workplace

In the study conducted at IBM, the focus was on what they called a 'break point analysis'. The break point was defined as the point at which difficulty managing work–life demands becomes so onerous that it is reflected negatively in workplace outcomes. The break point they used was when 50 per cent of the employees reported work–life difficulties. They found that the number of hours a person worked each week was the strongest predictor of the level of work–life difficulties experienced.

The most interesting finding was that for those without flexibility in when and where work is done, the break point was 52 working hours per week. However, for those with flexibility, the break point was 60 hours per week. *In other words, those who perceived they had flexibility were able to work an extra eight hours per week before they felt their work was negatively influencing their personal and family life.* In essence, flexibility enabled them to work 'an extra day a week' without creating additional work–life difficulty. For certain family characteristics, the results were even stronger. For women with pre-school children, the break point without flexibility was 32 hours per week; for those with flexibility it was 43 hours per week, an increase of eleven hours per week. This is an example of how flexibility contributes to the vitality of organisations, people, families and communities.

A similar study conducted in Australia also found that, for both men and women, those with higher levels of flexibility have a higher 'break point' in terms of the impact the hours worked have on their emotional wellbeing.

A growing body of research confirms the positive relationship between workplace flexibility and different aspects of workplace vitality. Findings show positive effects on employees' productivity, organisational commitment and engagement, retention, work attendance (lower absenteeism), morale, satisfaction and relationships with co-workers.

Benefits for fathers themselves

Research conducted in Australian organisations shows that fathers with high levels of flexibility also report higher levels of physical and psychological wellbeing.

What dads say about the work situation

'I must work in a very different place from most fathers. We have paid paternity leave and my boss, who recently became a new dad as well, took a couple of weeks off when his baby arrived. He encouraged me to do this as well, and even rang while I was off to have a chat about how things were going (and to keep me up with the gossip from work). This was good for me, as I picked up some of his responsibilities and got to develop some new skills. It was good for him too, because he saw that many of us were more capable than I think he thought we were. I now have regular chats with my boss about how things are going and the whole work environment is more flexible. The more I thought about it, I realised that some of the things we were doing at work – being more flexible, recognising diversity, teamwork and collaboration – were equally relevant at home. I even brought home one of the training manuals on conflict resolution and Jane and I looked at it together – using those "I" statements, though, can get a bit monotonous as we both know what each of us is trying to do!'

Julian, 40

'I have a great workplace – very different from what many men experience. I work in a manufacturing plant where all our work is organised in teams. We have our own work/family committee in our area. Seems a bit way-out there, doesn't it – a bunch of blokes with a work/family committee and our own budget! Well, I can tell you, it works. If someone has a family issue, say their wife is ill and he needs to be at home to care for the children, he comes to the group and we organise our work around it. He doesn't have to fill out forms, doesn't have to go to a supervisor, doesn't have to get permission from HR – we organise it ourselves. Or, if I want to work slightly different hours, as I did when we had Rachael – she was nine weeks premature and in intensive care for a long time. Belinda needed a lot of help – I came in to work early and left early for a period of about a month. The other blokes backed up for me.'

Ken, 34

'I found that I really had to work hard to get the kind of control over my job I needed to give me the flexibility to be at home at critical times. My supervisor is a woman and she doesn't have any children. I don't think she appreciated my need to be at home from around 5 p.m. Don't get me wrong, I am incredibly flexible with my hours – I come in early and am still prepared to put the odd hour in over the weekend when there is a breakdown. The thing that gets me is that my workplace expects me to be incredibly flexible when there is a work problem, but they don't seem to get it that there is a need for them to reciprocate when I have a family need.'

Jamie, 29

Many countries now have mandatory paternity leave for fathers of newborns, varying from two days to three weeks. Sweden, Italy and Norway even provide inducements for fathers to take parental leave.

Australia is starting to implement more policies that will increase the ways for families to better meet their work and caring responsibilities. Here are four factors that could improve the choices for fathers:

1 Unpaid parental leave for twelve months (available to both fathers and mothers)
   ★ This applies to the birth of a child or the adoption of a child under sixteen.
   ★ You need to have been employed in your organisation for at least twelve months.
   ★ Both parents can take leave at the same time under the following conditions: (i) it must be for a period of three weeks or less; and (ii) the joint unpaid leave must not start before the birth or adoption placement, and must not end more than three weeks after the date of birth or the day of adoption placement.

2 Paid parental leave (funded by the Federal Government)
   ★ Paid leave is available for eligible primary caregivers who have a baby or adopt a child.
   ★ Fathers who are primary caregivers can receive the parental leave benefit when their partner has returned to work.
   ★ The payment is for a maximum of eighteen weeks, at the national minimum wage.
   ★ Eligibility criteria include:
     – A work test: You need to have worked continuously for at least ten of the thirteen months prior to the birth, and worked for a least 330 hours during that period.

    – An income test: Your individual income must be less than $150 000 per annum.
    – You must not have returned to work.
    – You cannot also receive the baby bonus.

3 The right to request flexibility (e.g. part-time work; flexible hours, working from home)
    ★ This is a National Employment Standards Entitlement.
    ★ It applies to people who have had at least twelve months' continuous service.
    ★ This applies to employees who are either the parents of, or who have the responsibility for the care of, a child under school age, or a child under eighteen with a disability.
    ★ You need to make your request in writing, and employers must respond this request within 21 days.
    ★ Employers have a responsibility to thoroughly consider the request, but are able to refuse it on reasonable business grounds. Some of these reasons might be: a financial or work efficiency impact, an inability to redistribute work to existing staff, or an inability to recruit a replacement employee.

4 The right for men to claim discrimination on the basis of caring responsibilities, under the Sex Discrimination Act: workplaces should not discriminate against men who opt to take leave to care for their families or who adopt flexible work arrangements to share the care of their children.

If you don't enjoy workplace support, there are still things you can do to make work work for you.

What can you do?

There are two approaches you can take. The first is to focus on your personal responsibilities and the initiatives you could take to change your approach to your own job and career. The second is to become proactive in ensuring that your workplace becomes more father-friendly or father-inclusive.

Option 1: Take personal control of your work lifex

- Figure out what flexibility you want (e.g. flexible starting/finishing times or a compressed working week) and then check out your organisation's policies and your right to request flexible conditions.
- If you would like to have greater flexibility in how, when and where you do your work, and this is not currently available in your workplace, develop an argument for the flexibility you need and present this to your supervisor or workgroup. The key to achieving a positive outcome is to put the emphasis on mutuality – mutual responsibility for you and the organisation, and mutual benefits for you both as well.
- Analyse what your most important priorities are at work, then put more effort into these.
  (**Graeme:** One thing that I found worked for me was that I stopped attending what I considered to be unnecessary meetings; I figured that having one less person there would increase meeting efficiency as well.)

- Identify any non-essential work-related activities and eliminate them for a period of time (e.g. attending out-of-hours social activities). Say no to requests that are not central to your job (e.g. taking on a new project).
- Find ways to become more efficient at work. When we do this, we often find that we have too many unnecessary interruptions in our work lives (e.g. phone calls and emails), so try to work out a system for becoming more efficient at responding to all forms of communication.
- Adjust your expectations about what you are able to do. This might mean adjusting your career aspirations for a period of time. You will need to consider whether this will mean that you may be overlooked for career opportunities later. It is probably best to have a discussion with your supervisor or manager to make clear your intentions.
- Look for ways to have greater control over what you do. Do an audit of your situation every couple of weeks, to check how you are going with keeping your work in perspective.

Option 2: Take an active role in developing a father-friendly workplace

Here are a few policies and activities you could encourage management to put in place – or introduce yourself if you are in a position to do so:

- Encourage fathers to combine their jobs with their family commitments by introducing flexible work practices that fathers feel comfortable using (e.g. flexible hours; flexibility to attend medical appointments with their partner and/or child).

- Introduce paid paternity leave (e.g. for two weeks when a baby is born) and actively encourage fathers to use the leave. In company newsletters, congratulate new fathers who have taken leave.
- Ensure that fathers are included in any paid parental leave policy discussions or planning.
- Develop a forum for fathers to meet and openly discuss issues that affect their lives. Ensure that any family services include fathers.
- Introduce a Dads' Day at work, and encourage fathers to bring in their children.
- Encourage effective role models at the top by encouraging managers to take their fathering responsibilities seriously.
- Enjoy the benefits of employing men who have a strong commitment to family and community, as well as to their job and career.
- Frame your company as a father-friendly employer when recruiting, and in general advertising.
- Consider the different needs of fathers at different stages of their careers, and provide some career flexibility.
- Look for opportunities to affirm the role of fathers. For example, establish links with community organisations that focus on a positive approach to fathers.

Debates about work/family conflict and the impact work has on family life and vice versa go backwards and forwards. For some, the debate is about achieving work/life balance. This is a difficult concept to nail down – to understand just what it is and whether it is ever achievable. Balance also means different things to different people. When we ask groups of men what balance means to them, the answers vary – from issues to do with time, energy, relative influence (e.g. being around to influence their child's life) and their capacity to focus on the needs of their family, to an overall sense of peace and control where they feel they have choices and can directly influence how they spend their time.

Others believe that a father's time must either be totally invested in work, and not in home life, or the other way around. More enlightened workplaces now value the fact that their employees are committed to family life and place a priority on the father's contribution. This recognises that fathers can do both and still be successful at work. Recent research indicates though that this dual focus by fathers has inadvertently

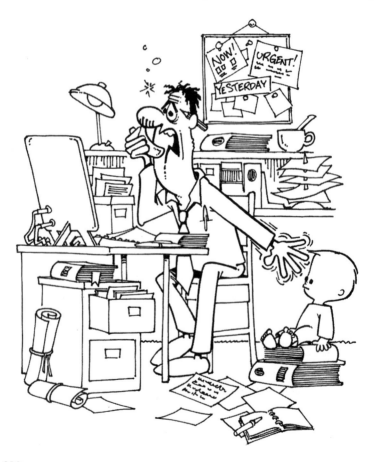

increased pressures on some fathers who 'do it all to have it all' – at the same time. This research also suggests that many men now consider the ideal man to be both successful as a financial provider, and as a father and partner.

In a recent study conducted in the US, 82 per cent of the sample of fathers agreed that family life made them feel happy and that this helped them to be a better worker; and nearly two-thirds agreed that involvement in their family life helped them gain knowledge that made them a better worker.

This has also been confirmed by recent research by Ellen Galinsky from the Families and Work Institute in New York. Her research shows that managing work and personal/family life is not a 'zero-sum game' where people give to one aspect of their lives and necessarily take away from the others. She found that those people with high-quality jobs and more supportive workplaces were more likely to walk in the door at home in a better mood and with more energy. Their work enhanced their family/personal life. This group was also found to be highly successful at work, hence Galinsky dubbed them 'dual centrics'.

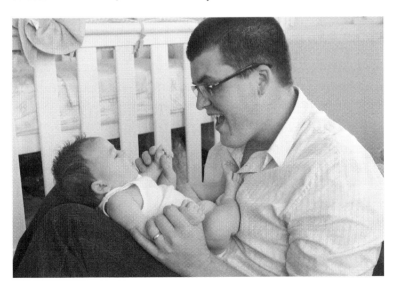

She also found that this group had a particular personal skill set that enabled them to perform effectively in both domains of their lives, e.g. being able to maintain strict boundaries between time working and time not working, and being able to focus on the immediate situation. When they were at home they were not thinking about work; instead, they were 'emotionally present'.

A challenge for us all!

Summary

★ The most common work–family challenges experienced by fathers are finding time for everything, switching off from work, and finding ways to make changes at work to improve this balancing act.

★ Doing an audit on how your time is spent is a good starting point. Once you're aware of your patterns, you can begin to make changes.

★ Some workplaces are becoming more supportive of fathers, but if this is not the case in your situation, then you can either change your approach to your own job, or work towards encouraging your workplace to become more father-friendly.

★ Research from around the world has shown positive outcomes for everyone – fathers, mothers, children and workplaces – when fathers are supported in the work environment.

A concluding comment

We began this book by talking about the excitement of being a father, and described it as a journey for life.

This book has been part of our own fatherhood journey. We have very much enjoyed sharing our thoughts and experiences with you. We have described the many ways you can be involved as a father and the multitude of changes that this can bring to your life. Fathers report that keeping focused on their child and staying connected with him or her through the many pathways of life is a richly rewarding experience. Being there for your child from the start, and being an equal member of your child's parenting team, are strategies that fathers find work for them and for their families.

Good luck!

Summary

Keep in mind:
- ★ You are important to your child
- ★ The relationship you develop with your child has a lasting impact
- ★ Being a dad is a lifelong journey – how you start is important
- ★ Your relationship with your partner does affect your child
- ★ Working as a team with your partner will make a difference

Things to do:

★ Regularly spend time alone with your child
★ Be curious about your child's development and discuss your questions with your partner
★ Put a priority on spending time with your partner to share the things that matter to you both
★ Use the TIMES diary (p. 193) to regularly check in on how you are spending your time – make adjustments if you need to
★ Focus on 'switching off' from work and 'switching' in at home
★ Look after your own health and wellbeing.

Authors' notes

Page 19 'The clear message from the research is that fathers matter and that mothers and fathers are both very important to their children': Lamb, M E (ed.), *The Role of the Father in Child Development*, 5th edn, Wiley, New York, 2010.

Page 20 'Research shows that babies become attached to both fathers and mothers – it depends on the parent responding sensitively to their needs ...': Lamb, M E & Lewis, C, 'The development and significance of father–child relationships in two-parent families', in Lamb, M E (ed.), *The Role of the Father in Child Development*, 5th edn, Wiley, Hoboken, NJ, 2010, pp. 94–153.

Page 30 'What you do with your children is influenced by many factors ...': Flouri, E, *Fathering and Child Outcomes*, Wiley, Chichester, UK, 2005. Lamb, M E (ed.), *The Role of the Father in Child Development*, 5th edn, Wiley, Hoboken, NJ, 2010.

Page 32 'The latest research affirms Harry's experience, telling us ...': Lamb, M E & Lewis, C, 'The development and significance of father–child relationships in two-parent families', in Lamb, M E (ed.), *The Role of the Father in Child Development*, 5th edn, Wiley, Hoboken, NJ, 2010, pp. 94–153.

Page 32 'While the process of influence for fathers is the same as for mothers ...': Lamb, M E (ed.), *The Role of the Father in Child Development*, 5th edn, Wiley, Hoboken, NJ, 2010.

Page 33 'For example, in one of the most widely cited studies, active involvement by a father in the pre-school years ...': Flouri, E, *Fathering and Child Outcomes*, Wiley, Chichester, UK, 2005.

Page 33 'In a recent Australian study, fathers with high levels of warmth and self-efficacy ...': Baxter, J & Smart, D, 'Fathering in Australia among couple families with young children', Occasional Paper No. 37, Australian Government, 2010.

Page 34 '... the quality of the father–child relationship is much more important ... than are the characteristics of individual fathers, e.g. the strength of their "masculinity".': Pleck, J H, 'Fatherhood and masculinity', in Lamb, M E (ed.), *The Role of the Father in Child Development*, 5th edn, Wiley, Hoboken, NJ, 2010, pp. 27–57.

Page 35 'Most infants form attachments to fathers and mothers at about the same age ...': Lamb, M E & Lewis, C, 'The development and significance of father–child relationships in two-parent families', in Lamb, M E (ed.), *The Role of the Father in Child Development*, 5th edn, Wiley, Hoboken, NJ, 2010, pp. 94–153.

Page 36 'The involvement of fathers during pregnancy ...': Plantin, L, Olukoya, A A & Ny, P, 'Positive health outcomes of fathers' involvement in pregnancy and childbirth paternal support: A scope study literature review', *Fathering*, vol. 9, no. 1, 2011, pp. 87–102.

Page 36 '... a partner with higher levels of psychological wellbeing...': Pleck, J H & Masciadrelli, B P, 'Paternal involvement by U.S. residential fathers: Levels, sources, and consequences', in Lamb, M E (ed.), *The Role of the Father in Child Development*, (4th edn), Wiley, Hoboken, NJ, 2004, pp. 222–71.

Page 37 'Research consistently shows that the quality of the relationship you have with your partner ...': Baxter, J & Smart, D, 'Fathering in Australia among couple families with young children', Occasional Paper No. 37, Australian Government, 2010.

Page 37 'Research conducted by John Gottman ...': Gottman, John, Gottman, Julie & Shapiro, A, 'A new couples approach to interventions for the transition to parenthood', in Schulz, M S, Pruett, M K, Kerig, P K & Parke, R D (eds), *Strengthening Couple Relationships for Optimal Child Development: Lessons from Research and Intervention, Decade of Behavior* Series, American Psychological Association, Washington, DC, 2010, pp. 165–179.

Page 38 'A common assumption is that workplace demands ...': Russell, G, & Hwang, C P, 'The impact of workplace practices on father involvement', in Lamb, M E (ed.), *The Role of the Father in Child Development*, 4th edn, Wiley, Hoboken, NJ, 2004, pp. 476–504.

Page 38 'Yet there has been surprisingly little research into the relationship between a father's involvement in his job ...': Russell, G & Hwang, C P, 'The impact of workplace practices on father involvement', in Lamb, M E (ed.), *The Role of the Father in Child Development*, 4th edn, Wiley, Hoboken, NJ, 2004, pp. 476–504; Haas, L & O'Brien, M, 'New observations on how fathers work and care: Introduction to the special issues – Men, Work and Parenting – Part 1', *Fathering*, vol. 8, no. 3, 2010, pp. 271–75.

Page 38 **'Findings are generally consistent in showing that higher levels of workplace demands …':** Russell, G & Hwang, C P, 'The impact of workplace practices on father involvement', in Lamb, M E (ed.), *The Role of the Father in Child Development*, 4th edn, Wiley, Hoboken, NJ, 2004, pp. 476–504.

Page 39 **'Recent US research findings also indicate that the level of work–life conflict…':** Aumann, K, Galinsky, E & Matos, K, *The New Male Mystique*, Families and Work Institute, New York, 2011.

Page 39 **'And recent Australian research shows that fathers with higher levels of negative work to family spillover …':** Baxter, J & Smart, D, 'Fathering in Australia among couple families with young children', Occasional Paper No. 37, Australian Government, 2010.

Page 42 **'Research shows that over 50 per cent of fathers make some adjustment to their work patterns as a result of having a child …':** Russell, G & Bowman, L, *Work and Family: Current Thinking, Research and Practice*, Department of Family and Community Services, Canberra, 2000.

Page 81 **'There is increasing evidence that classes directed at improving relationships during pregnancy …':** Gottman, John, Gottman, Julie & Shapiro, A, 'A new couples approach to interventions for the transition to parenthood', in Schulz, M S, Pruett, M K, Kerig, P K & Parke, R D (eds), *Strengthening Couple Relationships for Optimal Child Development: Lessons from Research and Intervention, Decade of Behavior* Series, American Psychological Association, Washington, DC, 2010, pp. 165–179.

Page 126 **'In one research study, mothers and fathers were observed interacting with their newborns: the fathers were as involved with and nurturing of their newborns as the mothers …':** Parke, R D, 'Perspectives on father–infant interaction', in Osofsky, J D (ed.), *The Handbook of Infant Development*, Wiley, New York, 1979.

Page 129 **'Research shows that, on average, few fathers spend a lot of time alone with their children …':** Russell, G, *The Changing Role of Fathers*, University of Queensland Press, Brisbane, 1983.

Page 131 'In the words of Professor Bryanne Barnett, "How parents look at and talk to their baby is crucial to a child's development ..."': Quoted from a paper given by Professor Barnett to a conference of the World Organisation for Early Childhood Education, Melbourne, July 2004. Professor Barnett is a Professor in the School of Psychiatry at the University of NSW and Director of Infant, Child and Adolescent Mental Health Services at the South Western Sydney Area Health Service.

Page 131 'Several studies indicate that infants with more responsive parents are more secure, more sociable and more independent ...': Lamb, M E (ed.), *The Role of the Father in Child Development*, 4th edn, Wiley, New York, 2004.

Page 132 'And research also shows that being confident and competent as a parent is critical for child outcomes.': Coleman, P K & Karraker K H, 'Self-Efficacy and Parenting Quality: Findings and future applications', *Developmental Review*, vol. 18, no. 1, March 1998, pp. 47–85.

Page 132 'As Michael Lamb ... has reported, 'The characteristics of individual fathers – such as their masculinity, intellect, or personality – are less influential in how children turn out than is the quality of the relationship ...': Lamb, M E (ed.), *The Role of the Father in Child Development*, 5th edn, Wiley, New York, 2010.

Page 132 'Fascinating facts about fathers' box: 'Parents – both fathers and mothers ...': Lewis, C & Warin, J, *'What good are dads?'*, *Father Facts*, vol. 1, issue 1, Fathers Direct, London, 2002.

Page 162 'Perhaps no aspect of child development is so miraculous and transformative as the development of a child's brain ...': Brotherson, Sean, 'Understanding Brain Development in Young Children' (2005), available at: http://www.ag.ndsu.edu/pubs/yf/famsci/fs609w.htm

Page 165 'Thinking that babies and toddlers are too young to be affected by domestic and family violence is a mistake ...': Factsheet Series – Children and Domestic and Family Violence, Queensland Centre for the Prevention of Domestic and Family Violence, September 2003.

Page 171 The ideas presented in **Chapter 8 'Connecting with your baby'** have benefited from the joint work Graeme has conducted with Peter Llewellyn-Smith.

Page 176 'Fascinating facts about fathers' box: 'Fathers who take on more responsibility ...': Lamb, M E & Lewis, C, 'The development and significance of father–child relationships in two-parent families', in Lamb, M E (ed.), *The Role of the Father in Child Development*, 4th edn, Wiley, New York, 2004.

Page 177 'According to Michael Lamb ... and Charlie Lewis ... "The establishment of attachment relationships between children and parents constitutes one of the most important aspects of human social and emotional development"': Lamb, M E & Lewis, C, 'The development and significance of father–child relationships in two-parent families', in Lamb, M E (ed.), *The Role of the Father in Child Development*, 4th edn, Wiley, New York, 2004.

Page 177 'Michael Lamb and Charlie Lewis point out that that there are four developmental phases in the establishment of attachment relationships ...': Lamb, M E & Lewis, C, 'The development and significance of father–child relationships in two-parent families', in Lamb, M E (ed.), *The Role of the Father in Child Development*, 4th edn, Wiley, New York, 2004.

Page 178 'Fascinating facts about fathers' box: 'Fathers can be just as sensitive and responsive ...': Lewis, C & Warin, J, 'What good are dads?', *Father Facts*, vol. 1, issue 1, Fathers Direct, London, 2002; Parke, R et al., 'Fathering and Children's Peer Relationships', in Lamb, M E (ed.), *The Role of the Father in Child Development*, 5th edn, Wiley, New York, 2010; Pleck, J H & Masciadrelli, B P, 'Paternal involvement by US residential fathers: Levels, Sources and Consequences', in Lamb, M E (ed.), *The Role of the Father in Child Development*, 4th edn, Wiley, New York, 2004.

Page 191 'We know from the research, though, that maintaining a high quality relationship with your partner has strong links with positive outcomes for children, and for you and your partner ...': Lamb, M E (ed.), *The Role of the Father in Child Development*, 4th edn, Wiley, New York, 2004, p. 280.

Page 198 'What can you do?' box: 'What you can do will depend very much on the type of job you have ...': text adapted from Galinsky, E, *Ask the Children: What Americans Really Think About Working Parents*, William Morrow and Company, New York, 1999.

Page 200 'Recent research shows that there are clear links between workplace support and the level of father involvement with their children ...': Hass, L, Allard, K & Hwang, P, 'The impact of organisational culture on men's use of parental leave in Sweden', *Community Work and Family*, vol. 5, no. 2, 2002, pp. 319–42.

Page 201 'Findings from an Australian study show that fathers who have supervisors who are more supportive of their needs are more likely to be highly interactive with their children ...': Ringland, P, *'The effect of organisational culture on father involvement'*, unpublished psychology honours thesis, Macquarie University, 2004.

Page 201 'In a study conducted at IBM ...': Hill, E J, Hawkins, A J, Ferris, M & Weitzman, M, 'Finding an extra day a week: The positive effect of job flexibility on work and family life balance', *Family Relations*, vol. 50, no. 1, 2001, pp. 49–58.

Page 202 'A similar study conducted in Australia ...': Hill, E J & Russell, G, 'Work and life: The business case', unpublished manuscript, 2008.

Page 206 'Option 1: Take personal control of your work life': Galinsky, E, *Ask the Children: What Americans Really Think About Working Parents*, William Morrow and Company, New York, 1999.

Page 209 'In recent research conducted in a range of organisations, close to 50 per cent of fathers said that their commitment to their job would be questioned if they used flexible work practices ...': Russell, G & Llewellyn-Smith, P, *'Working with men where they are: A report on workplace programs for men'*, unpublished manuscript, 2004.

Page 210 'Recent research indicates though that this dual focus by fathers has inadvertently increased pressures ...': Aumann, K, Galinsky, E & Matos, K, *The New Male Mystique*, Families and Work Institute, New York, 2011.

Page 210 'In a recent study in the US, 82 per cent of the sample of fathers agreed that family life made them feel happy...': Harrington, B, Van Deusen, F & Humberd, B, *The New Dad: Caring, Committed and Conflicted*, Center for Work & Family, Boston College, Boston, 2011.

Page 210 'This group was also found to be highly successful at work, hence Galinsky dubbed them "dual centrics" ...': Galinsky, E, et al., *Leaders in a Global Economy*, Families and Work Institute, New York, 2003.

Acknowledgements

The sequence of the authors' names does not imply superiority of role or contribution. This was a true partnership.

Tony: Writing this book with Graeme has been both exciting and challenging. As usual, with an enterprise of this kind, the outcome was achieved with the support of many. My partner, Anne, provided feedback and encouragement and she tolerated the time and obsession needed to complete the book. My girls have all been positive but are probably waiting for an opportunity to tell the world 'their version' of my parenting knowledge and skills. They often made comments like 'Did you tell them how often you served us broccoli?' and 'What about the time you embarrassed us in the shopping centre?' Regardless of my mistakes, they have developed into wonderful young women, and I'm proud of all of them.

I was lucky to have a wonderful mum and dad who provided not only love but also the inspiration and encouragement to work in my chosen field. It is my dad, in particular, who I would like to acknowledge as a role model; he demonstrated strong commitment to his partner and children until he passed away 18 years ago. I often think of what he taught me and how he cared, but I also thank him for what I did not experience as a child. He never showed me out-of-control anger. I never witnessed intolerance or racism in our home. He never made me feel bad – even when my behaviour was extremely challenging. He never made me feel unwanted or unloved. He never made me feel scared or frightened in his presence. What he did do was make me feel special and loved. I thank him for being my dad.

I also thank all the wonderful dads who have allowed me

to share a special time in their life. I hope this book will help new parents – especially new dads – as they start their incredible journey of fatherhood.

Graeme: My introduction to fatherhood began in 1972 and has not stopped since! I wish to acknowledge the contributions my wife Susan and our three children – Kirstine, Emily and Benjamin – have made to my learning and my opportunities; the pleasure I have experienced as a father, the continuing friendship I share with them and the support and love I receive from them. Having seven grandchildren – Steen, Leo, Kane, Tobias, Hugo, Otto and Elliot – and relating to their fathers and mothers, Terence and Emily, Damian and Kirstine, and Benjamin and Holly, has provided a fantastic new dimension to my fathering experience!

Thank you to Damian Hadley (with assistance from Kirstine and Leo) for allowing us to use the pie chart on page 115.

My experience as a father would not have been as deep and varied had it not been for Susan, my wife, who gently pushed me into being an involved father and who started out with the assumption that parenting was about having a team approach to sharing the pleasures and pains. Her love and support over a lifetime have been immeasurable.

I would also like to acknowledge friends and family, and other parents, who have shared their experiences and ideas with me over the years and provided support.

Finally, Macquarie University provided me with the opportunity to develop my interest in fatherhood and shared parenting.

Resources

A good starting point is to get to know the services available for parents in your local area. Most local councils have a services directory. Your doctor and local health services can also provide information. The resources listed here are some that new parents commonly find helpful.

Support services for parents

Keep all emergency numbers readily available – the fridge is a good display cabinet – including hospital, doctor, emergency services and 24-hour parent support lines.

Child Health Centres

All Australian states have free services offering assistance and support to families with children from birth to five years. The names of the services vary between states and include:

New South Wales	Child and Family Health Centres or Early Childhood Centres
Queensland	Community Child Health Centres
South Australia	Child Health Services
Tasmania	Child Health Centres
Victoria	Maternal and Child Health Centres
Western Australia	Child Health Centres
ACT	Maternal and Child Health Services
Northern Territory	Community Health Centres

Their services include:
- regular developmental screening
- information and support on breastfeeding and bottle-feeding, introduction of solids, sleep and settling, immunisation and a range of other parenting practices
- information about services available in your community
- referrals to specialist services.

Increasingly they also offer home visits, but the circumstances and number of visits also vary from state to state. Information about the service nearest to you can usually be obtained from your doctor or your local hospital. It will also be listed in your local phone book.

Australian Breastfeeding Association

This association provides support for mothers who are breastfeeding. There are support groups and trained breastfeeding counsellors in most areas of Australia. They can be contacted though the National Breastfeeding Helpline on 1800 686 268 (1800 mum 2 mum), and details of local services can be obtained from your Child Health Centre or hospital.

Family Support Services

These services provide a range of support for parents, including home visits, parenting groups, information and referrals. The services are free to parents with children up to twelve years of age in their care, though some also assist the parents of adolescents.

Parent Help Lines

The following services provide information and support 24 hours a day, unless specific hours are indicated.

New South Wales	Tresillian Parent Help Line 02 9787 5255 (Sydney metro area) or 1800 637 357 (local call cost from outside Sydney)
	Karitane Care Line 02 9794 1852 (Sydney metro area) or 1800 677 961 (local call outside Sydney)
Queensland	Telephone Information Support Service 07 3862 2333 (Brisbane metro area) or 1800 177 279 (local call cost from outside Brisbane)
	Parentline 1300 301 300 (operates 8 a.m. to 10 p.m.)
South Australia	Parent Helpline 1300 346 100
Tasmania	Parent Information Telephone Assistance Service 1800 808 178
Victoria	Parent Line 13 22 89 (operates 8 a.m. to midnight)
Western Australia	Family and Children's Services (08) 9272 1466 (Perth metro area) or 1800 654 432 (local call outside Perth)
ACT	Tresillian Parent Help Line 1800 637 357
Northern Territory	Parentline 1300 301 300 (operates 8 a.m. to 10 p.m.)

Websites

There are numerous Australian and international websites that provide information on most aspects of parenting. The Department of Families, Housing, Communities and Indigenous Affairs supports the Raising Children

Network and its website <http://raisingchildren.net.au>. The site includes a list of links to other parenting resources and services at <http://raisingchildren.net.au/services_support/services_support.html>.

The New Zealand Father and Child Society This Society is acknowledged as providing a respected national voice for fatherhood in New Zealand. It was created in 1998 to support local fathers' groups and organisations in setting up and running initiatives, as well as to improve access to information and improve communication between these groups. It helps represent fathers on a national level through the government's ongoing consultation process with the community. Website: <www.fatherandchild.org.nz>.

Fatherhood Institute Previously known as Fathers Direct, this is the UK's leading organisation promoting support for child–father relationships. Its mission is: 'To create a society that gives all children a strong and positive relationship with their fathers and other male carers, and prepares boys and girls for a future shared role in caring for children.' Website: <www.fatherhoodinstitute.org>.

We have reviewed many of the available websites and provide the following addresses of some of the better sites.

Safety

Kidsafe This is the trading name of the Child Accident Prevention Foundation of Australia, which focuses on providing information to prevent accidental injuries to children. There are offices in each Australian state and territory to provide up-to-date local information on safety issues for children. You will find links to all of the Kidsafe websites at: <www.kidsafe.com.au>.

NSW Fair Trading This site provides comprehensive and clear information for parents on a range of safety issues, including a very useful examination of baby products focusing on safety. Website: <www.fairtrading.nsw.gov.au>.

Similar sites for the other states and territories are:
- ACT Office of Fair Trading <http://www.ors.act.gov.au/community/fair_trading>
- Consumer Affairs and Fair Trading Tasmania <www.consumer.tas.gov.au>
- Consumer Affairs Northern Territory <www.consumeraffairs.nt.gov.au>
- Consumer Affairs Victoria <www.consumer.vic.gov.au>
- Consumer Protection Western Australia <www.commerce.wa.gov.au>
- Office of Consumer and Business Affairs South Australia <www.ocba.sa.gov.au>
- Office of Fair Trading Queensland <www.fairtrading.qld.gov.au>.

CHOICE The Australian Consumers' Association reviews and rates products and services, then publishes the results in its magazine and on its website. Of particular interest to new parents is the information on products for babies – the focus is on safety, quality and value. Website: <www.choice.com.au>.

Breastfeeding

We have already mentioned the Australian Breastfeeding Association as a resource. Its website also provides extensive information on all aspects of breastfeeding: <www.breastfeeding.asn.au>.

Child development

There are numerous websites with information on babies' development. We have reviewed a range of these and recommend the following. The Raising Children Network website lists many more.

Better Health Channel – Parenting This site provides user-friendly information on child development for children from birth to three years. It not only explains what is happening but provides options for parents to support babies' development. Website: <www.betterhealth.vic.gov.au>.

Brainwave A New Zealand site with excellent information on how your baby's brain develops and what enhances and inhibits brain development. It emphasises the importance of a caring, nurturing and stimulating environment, built on the 'responsive care' of your baby. Website: <www.brainwave.org.nz>.

Zero to Three A US site that provides easily accessible information corresponding to your baby's developmental age group. There is some great material on brain development. Website: <www.zerotothree.org>.

Books

There is no doubt that friends, relatives and service providers will recommend a number of books on pregnancy, birth and childcare. If you visit any bookshop you will find a range of books on offer. We have listed some that we think could prove helpful in your quest for extra information.

Pregnancy and birth

Eisenberg, A, Murkoff, H & Hathaway, S, *What to Expect When You're Expecting & What to Eat When You're Expecting*, 4th edn, Workman Publishing Company, New

York, 2008. This volume answers many common questions about pregnancy and includes a comprehensive guide on what's happening month by month. There is also detailed and easily understood information on diet during pregnancy, including lots of recipes and nutritional advice.

Morris, J, *Pregnancy, Childbirth & the Newborn*, rev. edn, Hinkler Books, Sydney, 2001. This book was first developed by the Childbirth Education Association of Seattle. Revised and updated by Dr Jonathon Morris, it provides a detailed account of the developing pregnancy, from conception to birth. It also covers the care of a newborn baby, and provides lots of detailed information.

Childcare

Lipsett, R, *Baby Care*, Finch Publishing, Sydney, 2012.
This book can inform you on all aspects of caring for your baby. It is very detailed, with good material on the concerns many parents have regarding the health of their baby. This book was written by a midwife with over 30 years' experience and is endorsed by the Australian College of Midwives.

Chilton, H, *Baby on Board: Understanding what your baby needs*, 2nd edn, Finch Publishing, Sydney, 2009. This book provides essential advice and explanations for parents, from the day of birth through the first months of babyhood, including reassuring medical information, a discussion of important issues that require parents' decisions, and a fascinating description of the evolutionary background to the needs of babies.

Fatherhood

Burgess, A, *Fatherhood Reclaimed: The making of the modern father*, Vermilion, London, 1997.

Lamb, M E (ed.), *The Role of the Father in Child Development*, 5th edn, Wiley, Hoboken, NJ, 2010.

Russell, G et al., *Fitting Fathers into Families*, Commonwealth Department of Family and Community Services, Canberra, 1999.

Vernon, D (ed) *Men at Birth*: Real stories from Australian men about the birth of their children, Finch Publishing, Sydney, 2011.

Index

Other Finch titles of interest

Raising Boys
Why boys are different – and how to help them become happy and well-balanced men (3rd edition)
ISBN 978 1876451 974

Raising Girls
Why girls are different – and how to help them grow up happy and strong
ISBN 978 1876451 592

Starting School
How to help your child be prepared
Sue Berne
ISBN 978 1876451 479

Up Downs
A fun and practical way to introduce reading and writing to children aged 2-5
Michelle Neumann & Kaye Forster
ISBN 978 1876451 806

Adproofing Your Kids
Raising critical thinkers in a media-saturated world
Tania Andrusiak & Daniel Donahoo
ISBN:978 1876451 875

Baby Care
Nurturing your baby, your way
Rhodanthe Lipsett
ISBN:978 1921462 306

A Handbook for Happy Families
A practical and fun-filled guide to managing children's behaviour
Dr John Irvine
ISBN 978 1876451 417

The Dad Factor
How father-baby bonding helps a child for life
Richard Fletcher
ISBN 978 1921462139

Shared Parenting
Raising your children cooperatively after separation
Jill Burrett & Michael Green
ISBN 9781876451721

Fathering from the Fast Lane
Practical ideas for busy dads
Dr Bruce Robinson
ISBN 978 1876451 219

Parenting after Separation
Making the most of family changes
Jill Burrett
ISBN 978 1876451 370

Stepfamily Life
Why it is different – and how to make it work
Margaret Newman
ISBN 978 1876451 523

Bully Blocking
Six secrets to help children deal with teasing and bullying
Evelyn Field
ISBN 978 1876451 776

Chasing Ideas
The fun of freeing your child's imagination
Christine Durham
ISBN 978 1876451 189

Fear-free Children
Dr Janet Hall
ISBN 987 1876451 233

Fight-free Families
Dr Janet Hall
ISBN 978 1876451 226

The Happy Family
Ken and Elizabeth Mellor
ISBN 978 1876451 127

Easy Parenting
Ken and Elizabeth Mellor
ISBN 978 1876451 110

ParentCraft
A practical guide to raising children well
(Second edition)
Ken and Elizabeth Mellor
ISBN 978 1876451 196

Your Child's Emotional Needs
What they are and how to meet them
Dr Vicky Flory
ISBN 978 1876451 653

Tricky Kids
Transforming conflict and freeing their potential
Andrew Fuller
ISBN 978 1876451 769

Life Smart
Choices for young people about friendship, family and future
Vicki Bennett
ISBN 978 1876451 134

Sometimes I Feel...
Samantha Seymour
How to help your child manage difficult feelings
ISBN 978 1876451 981

For further information on these and all of our titles,
visit our website: **www.finch.com.au**